Picking Up the Pieces

PICKING UP
THE PIECES

Moving Forward After Surviving Cancer

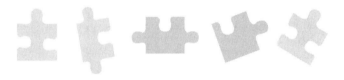

Sherri Magee, Ph.D. &

Kathy Scalzo, M.S.O.D.

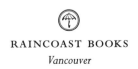

RAINCOAST BOOKS

Vancouver

Raincoast Books gratefully acknowledges the ongoing support of the Canada Council for the Arts, the British Columbia Arts Council and the Government of Canada through the Book Publishing Industry Development Program (BPIDP).

Edited by Barbara Pulling
Copyedited by Betsy Nuse
Cover and interior design by Teresa Bubela

LIBRARY AND ARCHIVES CANADA CATALOGUING IN PUBLICATION

Magee, Sherri
Picking up the pieces : moving forward after surviving cancer / Sherri Magee and Kathy Scalzo.

ISBN 10 1-55192-901-5
ISBN 13 978-1-55192-901-9

1. Cancer—Psychological aspects. 2. Cancer—Popular works.
I. Scalzo, Kathy II. Title.
RC262.M33 2006   362.196'994   C2005-905451-4

Raincoast Books
9050 Shaughnessy Street
Vancouver, British Columbia
Canada V6P 6E5
www.raincoast.com

Printed in Canada by Friesens.

10 9 8 7 6 5 4 3 2 1

To all cancer survivors, we wish you strength,
courage and grace throughout your recovery journey.

Contents

ACKNOWLEDGEMENTS

Throughout the five years it took for this book to evolve from an idea to these printed pages, we often felt the book had a voice and spirit of its own as ideas continually flowed and the right person or assistance would appear exactly when needed. Many people generously gave of their time, their support, their expertise and their stories. While we cannot name them all, we are forever grateful for their help and inspiration.

First we'd like to thank the survivors who participated in our research and who shaped the direction of this book. We thank them for sharing so much of themselves — their stories of triumph and troubled times, of beliefs shattered and new ones formed, and of paths taken that strengthened their recovery and ones that impeded it.

We owe a debt of gratitude to all the individuals — survivors, family members, health care practitioners and spiritual clergy — who participated in our interviews, questionnaires, focus groups and workshops. We send our heartfelt thanks to the survivors who read and tested this material and gave their feedback, invaluable insights as well as support and encouragement. A very special thank you to Angie MacDougall, Sally McLean and Gail Konantz, survivors who validated our work and provided us with immeasureable information as they read, edited and added to our book. And we extend a special thanks to members of three focus groups who helped develop the book with us: the Abreast in a Boat Dragon Boat Group — Brenda Hochachka, Kate Doyle, Sally McLean and Pat Cryder; the women at Hernando Island — Sherri Killam, Joni Killam and Louise Cecil; and the Young Adult Cancer Network Group — Jared, Anna, Christina, Patricia, and Vik.

For their assistance in turning our manuscript into this publication, we give our heartfelt thanks to our publisher, Michelle Benjamin, and the amazingly talented staff of Raincoast Books for taking a chance with two first-time authors. Their unending support, education and expertise are greatly appreciated. Thanks to our editors Barbara Pulling, for pushing us until the last minute and for making these pages sing, and Michelle Barker who nurtured us through early drafts and copious changes and contributed numerous ideas.

We are grateful to the authors whose work inspired and preceded ours: Dr. Rachel Naomi Remen (*Kitchen Table Wisdom; My Godfather's Blessings*), Dr. Michael Lerner (*Choices in Healing*), The National Coalition for Cancer Survivorship (*A Cancer Survivor's Almanac*), Dr. Wendy Schelessel Harpham (*After Cancer: A Guide to Your New Life*), Susan Nessim and Judith Ellis (*Cancervive: The Challenge of Life after Cancer*), Joan Borysenko (*Minding the Body, Mending the Mind*) and Lawrence LeShan (*Cancer as a Turning Point*), Glenna Halvorson-Boyd and Lisa K. Hunter (*Dancing in Limbo: Making Sense of Life after Cancer*) and Lance Armstrong (*It's Not about the Bike*).

We are grateful to William Bridges, for 25 years of research and writing on transitions and sharing his own personal story in *The Way of Transition,* Peter Senge, for creating a theory of change and learning that provides a framework for both individuals and organizations (*The Fifth Discipline; The Dance of Change*), Maria Perkins-Reed (*Thriving in Transition*) and Carol Adrienne (*When Life Changes or You Wish It Would*) for creating two practical and very readable books on the challenges of surviving and thriving during times of change and transitions.

Athlete and author Lance Armstrong *(It's Not about the Bike)* confirmed our direction, validated our work, and inspired us.

We'd like to thank fellow authors Sherrill MacLaren (*Braehead, Invisible Power*), Paula Jang (*Cleaning and the Meaning of Life*), and David Kuhl (*What Dying People Want*) who inspired us, answered our numerous questions over the years and guided us along each step of the way.

Technical support is invaluable while writing a book, and we'd like to thank Liz Tillson for transcribing countless interviews and volunteering much of her time to organize files and help out with whatever we needed.

We could not have written this book without the ongoing support of special friends such as Elena Crippen, who held our hands and kept us focused across the years, Marg McCuaig and Debra Dunn-Roy, who helped us through our very first attempts at a few chapters, and Janie Brown, a friend and professional associate who challenged us to 'go deeper,' and whose words rang in our ears as we continued to develop the book.

Sherri would personally like to thank: Sherrill MacLaren, my mentor, friend, confidant, and all around point person for every inquiry, doubt and excited moment she shared with me throughout the entire process; Sharon Smith-Swan, who shared my journey, offered invaluable advice and provided a sounding board for many of the ideas in this book; my loving friends Jan Keast, Jessie and Tara Hungerford, Ruth Andermatt, Linda Durham, Michele Green, Liz and John Seibold, Patricia Trottier and Gwyn Morgan for their gentle support, constant praise and belief in my ability to write a book that was greatly needed; my mother for always being proud of what I accomplish; and Katie, Terry, Jessie, Paddy and Danny Lanigan for occupying their father/grandfather while I was madly writing and needed time to gather thoughts, put pen to paper and meet deadlines.

Kathy would like to personally thank: Louise Cecil, who shared my vision, held my hand, and provided a nurturing, secluded place to write; Sherri Kilam, who walked miles of forest trails encouraging a budding writer; fellow writers Pat Pope — who always believed there was a book — and Joyce Statton who taught me to be patient with the process; Laurie Misshula, Ilona Fehre and Chris Cameron, who were always there with a cup of tea and a listening ear; Debra Sloan and the Wednesday night clay sculpture class for providing a creative outlet for my own healing; the faculty of Pepperdine University's MSOD program, who taught art and heart along with the science of planned change; my parents, brothers, and sisters for their constant love and emotional support (a special thanks to my five sisters, who held a 6:00 am prayer vigil the day Raincoast Books reviewed our book proposal); my sons Shane and Kalen Leech-Porter for their insights, alternative perspectives, willingness to be my sounding boards, and "you can do it, Mom" encouragement; my mother, Celeste Scalzo, who fostered within me a love of literature and whose death from cancer taught me more than words can say about acceptance, forgiveness and love.

And finally, to our husbands — Hugh and Colin — whose steadfast love, patience, understanding and support allowed us to bring this creative labour of love to life. They were encouraging from the very beginning and remained our greatest fans throughout the five years it took to go from an idea to a book. We thank them for all they gave and continue to give us each and every day.

— Sherri and Kathy, January 2006

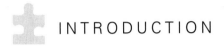 INTRODUCTION

Picking Up the Pieces

C *ancer survivor* — the very term triggers intense emotions. Reactions vary from *Hooray, I did it. I beat this horrible disease!* to *The label doesn't come close to capturing what my family and I have gone through.*

With the diagnosis of cancer, you are transformed from a person into a patient. Once your treatment is complete, you become a survivor. Certainly this new identity represents a triumph. Surviving is a reason for celebration. Survivors describe themselves as victors, graduates, or just plain lucky. As Susan, a three-year survivor of ovarian cancer, says, "I've made it through to the other side of a perilous minefield. Survivors understand exactly what I'm talking about when I say I'm happy to be alive."

But in practical terms, many people emerge tired and scarred from the battleground of cancer. Survivor, indeed: the survivor of a war that's been fought upon your very body and soul. In the words of Michael, a one-year survivor of lymphoma, "It was as if the silent enemy had chewed me up, spit me out and left me to fend for myself."

To survive the symptoms, treatments, and side effects of cancer is no easy undertaking. Whether you are still coping with the debilitating effects of therapy or you have no external physical evidence of the disease, research validates what you already know: cancer causes change. For some people the changes involve dietary adjustments, a new exercise routine or better stress management. But cancer can also lead you to question relationships, priorities, and even the meaning of life.

Once your cancer treatments have ended, you face the challenging task of picking up the pieces of your life and putting them back together again.

The response of many survivors can be summed up in one bewildered question: *Now what?* There are no set guidelines about where to go from here, no bridge from hospital to home. You could ask your oncologist for advice, but your follow-up visits will likely be focused primarily on physical concerns: side effects of therapy, changes in medication, the scheduling of further tests. That leaves little time for discussing the variety of changes you are experiencing. You may not even know how to describe them. All you know is that you're confused and that you feel out of sync with yourself and with others. As you grapple with what's happening to you, you often have the sense that you're all alone.

But you are not alone. We have written *Picking up the Pieces* to guide you through this difficult time. Although each person's story is unique, cancer survivors share similar concerns and face similar challenges. This book will help you navigate the healing process, although we believe that ultimately you are the expert on what you need. The recovery program you find in these pages will help you integrate who you were before cancer with who you are now. It will support you as you begin to acknowledge the changes that have occurred, grieve the losses, gain new insights into your experience and learn to live with the uncertainty of tomorrow.

Picking Up the Pieces is the first book to combine the inspiring voices of cancer survivors with a practical recovery process. Although we are not cancer survivors ourselves, between us we have spent more than 20 years working in the fields of cancer care and research, rehabilitative medicine, and change and transition management. In the course of our work, we have met hundreds of survivors from all walks of life. We developed this recovery program because so many survivors expressed a need for it, and many of them have generously shared the lessons they learned and the practical wisdom they gained in the hope that others will benefit. They were eager for others to understand that the end of treatment does not mean the end of the disease in a survivor's life. Rather, it is the beginning of learning to live with the experience of cancer.

Our interest in the field does come from personal experience. Sherri has had five people in her family diagnosed with cancer. Witnessing the impact of the disease inspired her to pursue a Ph.D. in interdisciplinary studies in order to understand the effects of cancer and its treatment on those who survive. For the past 15 years, she has designed personal cancer recovery programs for family, friends and clients and has trained physiotherapists, exercise specialists and personal trainers to work with cancer survivors in a variety of settings.

Kathy began her health-care career as an occupational therapist. She spent 10 years developing rehabilitation programs and services in acute care, long-term care and mental health settings. Pursuing a fascination with change and its impact on people's lives, she obtained a Master's degree in organizational development. For the past 20 years, she has worked as a consultant in the areas of personal, group and organizational change, designing processes and strategies in planning, problem-solving, conflict resolution, and change and transition management.

One of the most important things we've learned is that recovery happens one day at a time. It is a process of self-reflection, of sorting through life choices. Recovery is not so much about moving on as it is about moving through change. It's a time when you can decide to continue the things that contribute to your well-being and to abandon those that do not.

While the focus of treatment is on eliminating disease, the recovery phase is centred on healing the person. It is during recovery that survivors begin to shift their attention from illness to wellness. Healing is a journey of self-discovery that will almost certainly lead you into new territory. It will take you along uncharted paths, perhaps to places you never even knew existed. There will be sudden dips in the road, and the scenery is liable to shift unexpectedly. Your healing journey will require you to be open to change. But change is necessary to moving forward during recovery.

In presenting the recovery process, *Picking Up the Pieces* uses the metaphor of constructing a jigsaw puzzle. As a cancer survivor, you must reassemble the pieces of your life in order to feel whole again. Seeing all those puzzle pieces jumbled together can be overwhelming at first. But as you lay them out, sort through them, and find each of the four corners, a process emerges. You move out from the corners to frame in the puzzle's edges, then continue working towards the centre until eventually the entire picture unfolds.

We see the process of recovery as having four distinct phases: Inquiry, Discovery, Growth, and Reflection. Each phase allows you to recover a different aspect of yourself. By following our four-stage program, you will identify the changes you would like to make in order to embrace life fully — to live well after cancer. Our program also sets out two essential daily practices and offers questions that will help you to explore your abilities, thoughts, feelings, and desires as you move steadily towards regaining a sense of control over your life.

When time and patience are combined with determination, commitment and support, it is possible to 'assemble' even the most complicated puzzle. Whether you have just begun to pick up the pieces of your life or have been working through survivor issues for some time, we invite you to join us. It is our hope that this book will guide and support you in your healing process and you will emerge feeling whole again.

CHAPTER ONE

So, Where's the Party?

*"Bing, bang, boom, and ... I was out. Before my cancer I had never spent a
night in the hospital. Never had a stitch, never broke a bone; I'd hardly ever
had a shot. Then I was run through the wringer, and all of a sudden I was
cast adrift. That was a big shock."*

— Martin, 34 years old, testicular cancer, 1-month survivor

*"I felt so alone once treatment finished. The calls were not as frequent, the
casseroles and flowers stopped arriving at my door, the day-to-day
demands were resurfacing, and I just wanted to hide."*

— Janice, 41 years old, colon cancer, 3-month survivor

I t's your last day of treatment. You wave goodbye to hospital staff and walk
out those doors without looking back. It's done. You made it. All those
moments of terror and grief are behind you. Life will return to normal;
you'll resume your old routines. This is what you've been imagining for
months. That's why it comes as such a shock when you suddenly find yourself
riding an emotional roller-coaster, climbing giant mountains of joy and hope
only to hurtle down, without warning, to fear and disappointment. You didn't
expect to feel sad or scared. Everyone else is celebrating. Why aren't you?

Stepping back into everyday life after having faced a life-threatening
illness is not as simple as it sounds. Many survivors experience a tidal wave of
emotions once their treatment is over. These emotions can be conflicting, too.

At different times, you may feel overwhelmed, vulnerable, elated, exhausted, weak, relieved, anxious, grateful and unsure.

> *"I was so looking forward to a big celebration on my last day of radiation. My friends and family had called to say they were excited that it was almost over. I wore a new yellow blouse and brought chocolates for the nurses who had been so kind to me. My husband was waiting downstairs in the car ready to take me out for lunch. A few weeks earlier a woman had come to her last treatment wearing a graduation cap and I'd thought that was pretty cool, so I bought one for myself. But unfortunately, when I went to my last treatment, I had two new nurses. Then a woman came in, sat beside me and said she had just been told she had a recurrence. She was so angry. I thought, how can I be jumping up and down now? Needless to say, it took the wind out of my sails.*
>
> *"I had so many questions running through my head. Then the doctor came rushing in while I was getting dressed and said, 'You're in remission now, take good care of yourself.' I didn't even understand the word 'remission.' He was trying to be reassuring, but I was sad to see him go. I finished my treatment, got in the elevator and rode the four floors down. It seemed like an excruciatingly long time. I felt alone and disappointed. There was no chorus singing or band playing farewell. I felt a mix of relief and terror. I got to the car, saw my husband, and cried uncontrollably for half an hour."*
>
> — Nancy, 51 years old, breast cancer, 1-year survivor

Many survivors have a distinct last day of treatment, a day they look forward to for a long time. Others may need to continue with medications for years to come and do not have such a clear-cut finish line. The shape of your last day will depend upon the type and stage of the cancer you had, but it's a good bet that, like most survivors, you'll feel apprehensive as you resume everyday life.

It is not unusual to feel separation anxiety as your medical team withdraws its treatment support. As a patient, you became emotionally dependent on both the hospital staff and the treatment. Surgery, chemotherapy, radiation — these were your lifelines. The constant monitoring was a source of security;

the medical staff was your anchor. Suddenly you are cut loose. The treatments are finished. You don't need to come back for further care. These treatments had been keeping you alive, and now you have to believe that enough is enough. But is it? Without the protective bubble of treatment shielding you from the cancer, you may feel vulnerable or, even worse, abandoned.

> *"You're expected to go back into the world, supposedly cured, but nobody ever says you're cured. I started thinking: did they get it all? Should I have had more chemotherapy? Maybe I should get a topper-upper? Would the body I had trusted decide to grow a tumour again? The whole thing is so mysterious. I felt like I'd been cut loose to something unknown."*
> — Donna, 54 years old, ovarian cancer, 4-year survivor

THE SECOND HALF OF THE BATTLE

During treatment, patients develop a single-minded focus on beating the cancer. Many adopt a warrior stance, ready to fight the enemy with all they've got, doing whatever they must to stay alive. The treatment phase is filled with purpose and with hope that your efforts will carry you forward to win the battle. As Marion, a six-month survivor of breast cancer, puts it, "It was like the wagons had circled. My fears were all tucked deep inside, and I went into a rally-cheerleading kind of mode during treatment. Let's fight the good fight. Let the battle begin."

As a patient, your day is structured around cancer. You have appointments; there are friends, family and health care professionals standing by. But once treatment is complete, structure and focus give way to disorientation. Now your calendar is your own again. You feel disconnected and exhausted. Things slow down, and you are left alone with your thoughts and feelings. Finishing treatment turns out to be only half the battle. Your purpose must now switch from attacking the disease to healing from the experience.

> *"Once the treatment was finished and I wasn't in constant battle-mode, I fell apart. It's like a delayed reaction to just how horrible the experience really is, to feel that sick for so long, and to have*

your life under someone else's control. I felt so powerless."
— Cindy, 33 years old, lymphoma, 3-year survivor

UNEXPECTED CHANGES

Cancer treatment is a double-edged sword: it destroys the cancer, but it leaves you damaged. The cancer cells may be localized to a specific organ or system of the body, but treatment affects the whole person: heart, mind and spirit. Chemotherapy, radiation, and surgery can leave you struggling with a variety of short- and long-term side effects that influence recovery. While some survivors move on with hardly a backward glance, others are profoundly aware of the changes, losses and lessons that have come into their lives with cancer. In the wake of their illness, many are left on their own to identify, understand and learn to cope with these.

"After treatment finished, there was nothing, just the quiet. There was a lot of fear in that quiet. There was also the exhaustion and pain, which seemed to increase with time. I was so anxious for the doctors to get control of my cancer cells, I never thought about what would be left in the aftermath of treatment. While I was glad to have an aftermath to deal with, the side effects have become more of an issue the longer I survive."
— Doreen, 50 years old, breast cancer, 4-year survivor

Side effects are not just physical, though the physical ones might be the most immediate. Survivors identify change on four levels: physical, emotional, spiritual and social.

Physical Change
Some of the physical issues you may be confronting include fatigue, chronic pain or numbness, sexual dysfunction, and disfiguring scars. You might be unprepared for the new reality of incontinence, erectile dysfunction, early menopause, weight gain or loss, and mouth or teeth problems. Maybe you lost a breast. Maybe you gained a colostomy bag or an artificial voice box. It all means you must adjust to a new physical reality after cancer.

Emotional Change

When you wake up in the morning now, you don't know whether you're going to feel happy and grateful, or sad and teary. Some days you're depressed, angry and anxious. You can't concentrate; the smallest things overwhelm you. Your confidence level has plummeted. You don't trust your body any longer. You wonder whether you should talk to someone about how you're feeling, but you're not sure what person to approach.

Above all, there is the fear and uncertainty. Having cancer means facing the unknown trajectory of this disease, the prospect of side effects from the treatments and the possibility of death. Even though the doctors have told you that you're in remission, you can't help but worry: Will the cancer come back? How will I handle this state of constant insecurity? The fear of recurrence is heightened during the first year after treatment, and though its intensity does decrease over time, that fear seldom completely disappears. Follow-up doctor visits, yearly anniversary dates and the death of a fellow survivor are its most common triggers.

Spiritual Change

You may feel physically recovered, yet find that your spirit is still in the process of healing. This is a time when profound questions arise and refuse to be pushed aside: *Why did I get cancer? Why did I survive? What does my life mean?*

You might feel compelled to make sense of what has happened to you, to review your life and perhaps choose to live differently, to find new meaning or direction. For many there is a significant shift in awareness and a deep sense of connection to others. Some survivors speak of a renewed spirituality and a strengthened relationship with God, their community and/or nature. Others question their spirituality, the strength of their faith or the lack of it.

Social Change

Now that you've survived cancer, you may be unprepared for the changes that have occurred in your relationships with friends, family members, and colleagues, even with your spouse. While you were in treatment, your support team had clearly defined roles to play. They stood by your side, rubbed your back, brought you soup. But now they need to resume their lives.

Many relationships are strained by the demands of treatment, and recovery often takes longer than anyone expects. This can be frustrating and disappointing for everyone. Your family and friends may harbour unexpressed fears for your survival. You are struggling with your own fears and anxieties but feel uneasy about burdening anyone with your troubles. And so you suffer silently, when what you need most is to talk to someone about your feelings.

SURPRISE ENDINGS

Once treatment was over, you thought there would be time to take a deep breath. Instead, you find yourself facing some unforeseen challenges.

> *"Had someone told me, I wouldn't have believed that life after cancer could be more difficult in many ways than life with cancer. I thought I was done with cancer, but I have been dealing with the side effects of cancer and its treatments for over a year now."*
>
> — Randy, 37 years old, lymphoma, 1-year survivor

We will talk more about the nature of change at various points in this book, but what's important to acknowledge is that there is a disparity between what you expected from recovery — a smooth landing — and what you got: a crash. In fact, it is this disparity that creates the space in which you find yourself after treatment. We call it the Void.

ENTERING THE VOID

Once treatment ends, you arrive in the lost land between patient and survivor. You're not really sick anymore, but you don't trust your health, either. Survivors describe this as an in-between place, limbo, a weird nothingness, a neutral zone.

> *"When I left my last treatment, I had the image of coming out of a dark tunnel into a bright light. You can't really see anything clearly, and you're disoriented. It was like coming out of a movie into the sunshine,*

not knowing where I was. I had endured a hardship, I'd been through a long
process, and now I was left somewhere strange and unfamiliar. I didn't
know how I was going to move forward from there."
                    — Fiona, 42 years old, bladder cancer, 1-year survivor

There are no maps to help you navigate the Void. It is an empty land that all
survivors must cross, and the only instructions you get are "Wait and see."
Any progress you make comes hard-won, through trial and error. It's as if
you are suspended in a pool treading water, not knowing which way to
swim: back to the safe, shallow end you came from, or forward into the deep
unknown.

But frightening as it may be now, forward is the only way out of the
Void. To advance, you must make the transition from the past to the
unknown future. As human beings we naturally seek what is familiar to us.
It is scary to face down the unpredictable and embrace change. Yet that is
what you must do when you enter the Void. This is a time of feeling lost and
directionless, a time of not knowing. In their book *Dancing in Limbo*, cancer
survivors Glenna Halvorson-Boyd and Lisa Hunter explain: "We felt lost in
the most familiar places — home and work and play — among our most
familiar people — family and friends. Nothing seemed the same, and of
course, it was not, because we were not the same." (1)

The landscape of this post-treatment no-man's-land is as varied as the
people who travel its peaks and valleys, but in our work we've found eight
emotional landmarks that survivors may pass along the way. You might
encounter all of these at different times during your recovery, or you may
become familiar with only one or two. Whatever the case, all of these landmarks are common to cancer survivors who have walked this path already.

Filling the Calendar

Now that your carefully scheduled treatments are over, you find yourself
craving a new daily routine in order to regain control over your life. Maybe
this means adhering to a strict new diet and exercise regime, joining a support group or trying various complementary medicines. Maybe it means
resuming your former activities. Your attitude might mirror that of Stuart, 61

years old and a four-month survivor of prostate cancer: "I just want a pre-dictable pattern to my life again, something that will give me peace of mind. Otherwise I feel like I'm floundering."

It's Not Fair

You are caught up in resentment of how the cancer has left you: physically changed, fearful of a recurrence, and saddened at having to deal with it all. You feel as if you've lost your way in this formless space of recovery.

> "At the end of ten months, I felt powerless to change what had happened to me. I'd had a double mastectomy, my hair grew back thin and stringy, I had nightmares about dying almost daily and I often woke up in a cold sweat. I was not able to focus for any length of time and my thoughts felt scattered. I was depressed and had big mood swings. I was not healing."
> — Deborah, 38 years old, breast cancer, 10-month survivor

I'm Glad to Be Alive

You feel grateful for each day, for each moment of life you have been given after your brush with death. Instead of planning too far ahead, you live one day at a time.

> "I'm so happy I'm feeling good now. I spend time every day thanking God. I get up and go, Wow, yesterday was great and today I feel good. I sit in the morning drinking my coffee with my cat curled up on my lap, not caring if she leaves her white hair all over my black housecoat. I'm just grateful to be alive."
> — Bridget, 49 years old, colon cancer, 1-month survivor

It's My Life

No one warned you recovery would be this hard. You're not receiving the help you need, and it angers you that no one has the answers you want. You're fed up with the lack of control over your life, so you rebel with alcohol, drugs, an unhealthy diet and little sleep. You live fast, not stopping to consider the cause of your pain. *To hell with the cancer* is your attitude.

You survived, didn't you? You deserve to live the life you want.

> *"I felt betrayed by what had happened to me. I went on a do-what-I-want rampage for a while. I drank too much wine, I abused prescription drugs and I ate whatever I wanted. If I was going to die soon, I wasn't going to deny myself anything."*
>
> — Anne-Sophie, 43 years old, breast cancer, 9-year survivor

The Black Hole

You don't understand why, but you feel a big hole in the pit of your stomach. Your days are sad and lonely, your nights sleepless. The fear of recurrence runs through your head repeatedly. You are overwhelmed by all of the changes you've had to undergo.

> *"I am still in what I call 'numb-numb land' most of the time. I'm in that place between living and curling up in a ball, trying to protect myself. But I don't even know what I'm protecting myself from. I just can't seem to move."*
>
> — Daphne, 51 years old, colon cancer, 2-month survivor

Getting Back on the Horse

You've always heard that if you fall off a horse, you need to get right back on, before fear overtakes you. As soon as you can, you jump back into everyday activities, frantically trying to re-establish old routines at home and work, and with family and friends. Some survivors find this the best way to live with uncertainty. But many discover that charging back into the old way of life isn't as easy as they had expected — nor as fulfilling.

> *"I was so eager to prove to everyone — and to myself — that nothing had changed in my life. I went straight back to my job after treatment ended, but after working for a short while I lost enthusiasm for the job I'd always loved."*
>
> — Michael, 42 years old, lymphoma, 6-month survivor

Catch Me If You Can

You feel compelled to make up for all that lost time spent in treatment by doing as much as you can. You start various creative projects, or maybe you go on an extended holiday. You embark on a new lifestyle that turns your family upside-down. Whatever it is, you make sure you run as fast as you can, to live the life you want in whatever time you have left.

> *"I wanted to cram everything into the next week. My days were full, full, full; everything was in motion. I didn't want to waste a minute. I didn't stop to think about what I was doing, I was just going. I joined an art class, saw friends daily for a walk, and started going to yoga. I was gasping for air, and grasping for lost time."*
>
> — Sin-Yu, 54 years old, ovarian cancer, 4-month survivor

Who Asked You?

Everybody seems to have advice for you about how to stay healthy: you're drinking too much coffee, eating too much sugar, not exercising enough, not sleeping enough. You should be taking a yoga class, you should be meditating, have you heard about the latest research on stress, have you remembered to relax? People mean well with their advice, they really do, but that doesn't mean it isn't confusing and often annoying to hear. And personal advice is the least of it. Magazine articles about health and cancer abound. Internet sites have multiplied by the thousands. It is hard to listen to your own mind and body amid the cacophony of information that surrounds you.

> *"I read so much conflicting advice that I started to doubt myself. What if I've chosen the wrong strategy? What if I'm missing something? I couldn't be sure of anything anymore."*
>
> — Stan, 63 years old, melanoma, 1-year survivor

NORMAL DOESN'T FIT ANYMORE

All the survivors we've encountered in our work expect at first that their lives will get back to normal, even though they've just survived a disease and treatment that makes returning to their old selves almost impossible. This is the wishful thinking cancer survival engenders: that after treatment ends, you can pick up your life where you left off.

If you ask your doctor what normal is, he or she will probably focus on the disease process. Dr. Graham Smith explains: "We say to our patients, 'You're normal because you don't have signs of cancer left. Now you're free to go about your business and live the rest of your life.' Some hear that to mean they will be the same as they were before their diagnosis. But many know they are not the same person they once were. Compared to how they were before the treatment, many are profoundly and fundamentally changed." (2)

Acknowledging change and worrying about recurrence make the task of getting back to normal a complex one for cancer survivors. In fact, the real issue is not to get back to normal, but to find out what normal is for you now. It is normal to alternate between feeling an incredible sense of loss and having a renewed appreciation for the simple things in life. It is normal to keep looking over your shoulder to compare who you were before cancer with who you are now. It is also common for your idea of normal to be different now from what it was pre-cancer.

If you run into friends and ask them, "How are things?" they will likely talk about their hectic lives. For many people, normal means being stressed out, overwhelmed, and exhausted, with little relaxation time. If this was your definition of normal before cancer, is it really what you want to return to? People who long to get back to normal may not realize that what they're yearning for is something completely different.

It is also typical to worry that you're not normal. As a non-smoker, Beth was shocked to be diagnosed with lung cancer. She speaks about how difficult it was to resume her previous roles without any reassurance that her mood swings during this time of transition were natural and to be expected.

"I began to take on more of my share of the work at home and at the office. But everything was an effort. I was so grateful to be alive, but even my kids and their littlest squabbles drove me crazy. I'd yell and then I'd feel guilty. And at work, the problems people complained about all seemed so trivial. I seemed to fluctuate between thinking nothing was a

big deal to worrying that everything was a tragedy, I lost my bearings.
I felt upside-down. I was struggling to try and just be normal again, but I
was no longer sure what that meant."

    — Beth, 34 years old, lung cancer, 6-month survivor

Family and friends are just as eager for life to return to their view of normal.
If you think they're watching you, you're right. Everyone wants reassurance
that you are behaving the way you always did, returning to the routines
you've always followed.

    Leona had a double mastectomy. Her sister, Patricia, travelled across the
country to support her during the surgery. Patricia returned later for a visit
and was delighted to see Leona back to her old self. Leona's response was
more ambivalent:

"It's strange, because there is still a part of the old person left inside me,
yet I can never really go back to being that same person. I didn't want to
return to work as I knew it. I didn't know where to go next. I didn't know
what I wanted to do with my life. I finally stopped to ask these questions,
and it was a hard place to be in. Once you've had an experience with can-
cer, it shapes who you are and how you see the future."

    — Leona, 44 years old, breast cancer, 6-month survivor

DISCOVERING A NEW NORMAL

As a survivor of cancer, you face the task of picking up the pieces of your life
and trying to fit them into some new way of living. Your goal is to move
beyond surviving to start engaging in life more fully. You know this won't
happen overnight. But where do you start? How do you find a new normal?

    To discover and define your own new normal, you will need time,
courage, and a willingness to explore change. You've gone through many
changes in your experience with cancer, and the prospect of even more
change may — understandably — make you nervous. But keep reading.
What you discover might be more reassuring than you'd expected.

CHAPTER TWO

Having New Eyes

"To look at me, you'd think nothing remarkable had happened. From the outside, my world looks pretty much the same as before the cancer. I'm still a busy homemaker, actively involved with the kids' school and sports activities, and I'm a regular volunteer at our church. But inside, my thoughts, attitudes and feelings have completely changed."

— Liane, 38 years old, leukemia, 1-year survivor

"Many people with cancer come to divide their lives in half: before and after cancer. You are never the same again."

— Sandra, 42 years old, ovarian cancer, 2-month survivor

At the heart of every change is a paradox. As one thing falls away, something new is created to take its place. The bud becomes the flower that blooms. The caterpillar is transformed and the butterfly ascends. From birth on, we are part of a constantly changing, never-ending flow of experience. Just as our bodies develop and change with time, so does everything else about us: our thoughts and emotions, our relationships, our finances, our health. Change is a basic ingredient of life.

But with change comes uncertainty, an unpredictability that can destabilize us and disrupt our lives. Change requires us to behave or respond in new and different ways, which can be uncomfortable. Change may, and often does, require having to give something up. So, not surprisingly, our initial reaction to change can be to ignore it, avoid it, or resist it at all costs.

Change — which may well be a blessing — can at first feel more like a curse.

Because change is often precipitated by a particular event, we tend to view change itself as something finite, with a beginning and an end. Once the event is over, we want to return to the status quo, to get on with our lives as quickly as possible. This idea of getting back to normal contains a hidden message: we are expected to act as if nothing has changed.

We are always changing; that isn't something we can control. But what we can control is our reaction to change. Most of life's changes are gradual and cumulative, as opposed to being traumatic and transformative. When a traumatic event such as a life-threatening illness occurs, we call upon our coping skills and behaviours to help us address the immediate crisis. But our ordinary coping behaviours may be inadequate to deal with the magnitude of change that a crisis can bring. We can choose to be bitter, angry, and depressed; indeed, many people do, without even realizing it. Or we can learn strategies that will develop our stamina, give us a robust attitude towards change, and teach us the flexibility that is necessary for swimming with the ebb and flow of life's currents.

CANCER CAUSES CHANGE

As we progress through life, we experience times of transition that we learn to expect and come to understand. But the changes caused by cancer are usually unanticipated and always uninvited. Many survivors experience change overload — too many changes happening simultaneously. Although some of these changes may be relatively minor, cancer also causes profound change that requires both an internal shift in values and aspirations and an external shift in behaviour.

Many of us view change from an either/or perspective: it either helps us or hinders us. Change that is beneficial adds something positive to our lives, we believe. It takes us in a direction we are pleased to go. Change that hinders us upsets our lives. It forces us to alter our plans and rethink our expectations and it leaves us feeling disoriented and deceived. The changes that result from cancer, however, are not so easy to categorize.

As difficult as treatment can be, some survivors see cancer as a catalyst that prompts them to make significant changes in their lives, from simply taking time to appreciate each new day to learning to take better care of themselves. Cancer becomes a harbinger of personal growth.

> *"Before my cancer, I was often afraid to try new things or do something different. But I just began singing lessons, and this summer I'm off on my first kayak camping trip. I have a chance at living again, and I try to take a moment every day to really appreciate just being alive."*
> — Joshua, 24 years old, testicular cancer, 2-year survivor

A different aspect of change involves the pressure you might put on yourself to do something profound. You have been spared; therefore, you think there must be something special you are supposed to do. After all, look at Lance Armstrong: he had cancer and then went on to win the Tour de France several times. *What am I going to do?* you ask yourself in that tone of voice that suggests a dare.

It doesn't help when other people project their expectations onto you. Friends and family members may mean well when they ask, "What big things are you going to do with your life now?" But in fact they are contributing to the unrealistic expectation that you must do something impressive because you've survived cancer.

> *"A friend recently asked me, 'So what amazing feats are you going to accomplish since you're better?' She doesn't understand that I've just completed the most amazing feat of my life!"*
> — Patricia, 36 years old, breast cancer, 3-month survivor

Maybe a vision of your new life will magically appear, and you will find your way to a magnificent future accomplishment. But what if this grand-scale change never happens? Does that mean you've failed somehow or missed something? Is this the only kind of change that has value?

Actually, the biggest change challenging cancer survivors is also the one that is easiest to miss. The quiet change happening deep within your very being is the tiny puzzle piece that hides beneath the others, blends in, and doesn't seem to matter. And yet it makes the most difference of all.

The French author Marcel Proust expressed it most poetically: "The real voyage of discovery consists not of seeking new landscape, but in having new eyes." (1) Recovery from cancer requires, quite simply, a willingness to work with change. If you can accept the reality of change in your life, you are already seeing the world with new eyes.

TRANSITION: THE PLACE BETWEEN

If change involves letting go of one trapeze bar in order to grab hold of another, the space in between — where you're left hanging in mid-air — is called transition. Change is the event that rocks your life; transition is the passage, the time when you must learn how to be this new person that has been forced upon you. Transition means coming to terms with the new environment in which you find yourself. For cancer survivors, this requires learning how to navigate the Void.

"Change can happen anytime," writes William Bridges in *The Way of Transition*, "but transition comes along when one chapter of your life is over and another is waiting in the wings to make an entrance." (2)

Every transition begins with an ending: divorce, a change in employment, serious illness, the death of a loved one. Such events disengage you from life as you have known it. Change disrupts the internal systems you have developed to reinforce your sense of self, your beliefs and assumptions, your roles and dreams for the future. Whether the change is gradual or sudden, it places you in unfamiliar territory. You feel lost. Your life no longer makes sense, or perhaps it isn't as fulfilling as it used to be. In transition, a person finds him- or herself somewhere between giving up the old and coming to terms with the new. The past is gone, but the future is not yet here.

These feelings can be very confusing. Perhaps you were already dissatisfied with your life and you welcome the prospect of change. But what if your old life was full of meaning? You might feel uneasy at the thought of tossing it all out the window, as if it had suddenly lost its value. And of course, it hasn't. During any transition, it is important to honour your past. What served you well once may not serve you now, but that doesn't mean it wasn't useful in its time. As Carl

Jung wrote, "We cannot live the afternoon of life according to the programme of life's morning; for what was great in the morning will be little at evening, and what in the morning was true will at evening have become a lie." (3)

During transition, much of our external life might look the same. We may do the same work, live in the same house, shop in the same neighborhood, and keep the same friends. Yet internally, we are encountering unfamiliar parts of ourselves. As Irene, 29 years old and a six-year survivor of lymphoma, describes it, "No one could guess how much and how quickly I was changing. They all saw the same old Irene, but on the inside my life had been turned upside-down."

At its heart, transition is as paradoxical as change. There is a gap between the current state of our life and what we want. This gap may be filled with tension and discomfort, but these feelings provide the impetus for us to pursue new opportunities. As William Bridges acknowledges in *The Way of Transition*, the very things we now wish we could hold onto were themselves originally produced by changes. He stresses that it is not change most people resist, but rather the pain and discomfort of the adjustment period of transition.

Cancer's Double Whammy

While change triggers transition in everyone's life, cancer survivors experience two world-shaking, back-to-back transitions. Understanding transitions, along with learning to cope and adapt to the changes they bring, is a process that continues throughout your life.

Your life before cancer was filled with ongoing change, dotted by high and low points, which have triggered transitions in the past. The first major cancer-related transition occurs when you are diagnosed with cancer. In this transitional phase, you enter the structured medical environment, are labelled a *patient*, given a file number, and taken through treatment. It is during treatment that you lose your sense of identity, of control, and of meaning. The immediacy of the present precludes any thoughts of the future. No words can capture the depth of angst, fear and worry that are characteristic of the time spent in treatment. For many, the potential of death associated with cancer causes it to tower over previous life traumas.

A second transition begins on the last day of treatment when you receive the new label of *survivor.* The completion of treatment triggers entrance into a post-treatment Void, which is the beginning of the transition from survivor back to a healthy individual. This second transition is all the more cruel for being so often unexpected. It is during this time that you address the side effects of treatment and try to find a new normal. You are learning how to heal, while at the same time trying to resume your daily life. The second transition ends when you have defined a new normal for yourself and feel able to put your cancer experience in context with the other significant transitions in your life.

Picking Up the Pieces focuses on the second transition, introducing a process that will help you heal by guiding you across the Void. You will learn how to explore new choices in order to live well with the experience of cancer.

In the Bardo

It is often only in retrospect that people can acknowledge the power and impact of a crisis. While you are caught in the middle, it is nearly impossible to see any potentially positive outcome. Part of the reason for this is that North American society has few rituals to assist people through times of crisis, let alone mark the time between endings and new beginnings. In the Tibetan tradition, there is a name for the space between lifetimes — the place you inhabit after you have left your physical body but have not yet been reincarnated into a new one. You are said to be in the bardo.

In her book *Navigating the Future,* psychologist Mikela Tarlow writes: "There is little support in our society for such periods. Secretly, people are horrified when they hear you say, 'I don't know,' or, 'I'm not sure.' They immediately offer you advice and referral to their favorite 'fixer-uppers' so you can quickly get out of your confusion. Imagine if people began to respond to our vagueness by saying, 'How lucky, you're in the bardo, take your time, don't even try to figure it out.'" (4)

By acknowledging that transition not only exists but is a valuable time of learning and reassessment, we dispel the fog that obscures our view of the present situation. The puzzle of our life remains, and putting it together is part of what living is all about. How do you find your way back to your old life? How do you find a way to embrace your new life? Answering these questions is part of the process of change and transition.

THE CHANGELESS CORE

Whether we are aware of it or not, deep within us we have psychological strengths and resources, fundamental values and a sense of purpose, all of which serve as True North on the compass we rely upon to make life decisions. Even though this point may be hard to locate, it's there, and it's unshakable. Think of it in whatever way works for you: your anchor, your centre, your lifeline, the force that pulls you forward. In psychological terms, it is known as the core self. Your core self sees you through the highs and lows of life as you progress forward. Your core self is the unchanging part of you that has seen you through difficult times of change in the past and is helping you through this one.

In her book *When Life Changes or You Wish It Would,* Carol Adrienne writes, "There was both a comfort and a sadness in the realization that the things I used to ache for 30 years ago, I still ache for. The things I cared about are still the things I care about. I still try to live near water. I still have too many books. I might learn how to use gadgets like a Palm Pilot, but in the things that really matter to me, I always knew what I needed to know." (5)

Sally, a three-year survivor of melanoma, describes the strong connection she feels to her core: "Nobody else has handled, or will handle, their cancer experience in the same way as I am doing it. Everyone is unique. My core self affects how I look at life and how I live it. It is what got me through my illness, and it is there guiding me as I go about recovery."

Our core self remains whole and untainted by even the most horrific experiences. It links us to our past, and it influences how we handle adversity. When fear arises, our core self helps us hold firm. When we identify and listen to our core self, we experience healing in all aspects of life. Honouring your core self can allow you to live well despite cancer-related limitations.

"I held on tightly to my core, my sense of who I was, so as not to become the disease. I was not the breast cancer. I was Manuela, a woman with breast cancer."

— Manuela, 45 years old, breast cancer, 2-year survivor

Maintaining a connection to our authentic self reminds us that while much may have changed in our circumstances, our essence remains the same. Your core self may not always be easy to find. It may be so deeply buried, calling with such a faint voice, that you tell yourself it doesn't exist. You may have to chip away thick layers of doubt and fear to reach it. Everyone begins their cancer experience from a different place, and everyone has different coping skills, strategies, and levels of support. But we can all create and maintain personal stability by asking ourselves *What has changed? What has stayed the same?*

COPING VERSUS ADAPTING

Most people respond first to a life-changing event by trying to cope. Coping is the set of actions and behaviors we call upon in response to a stressful situation. When you find yourself dangling from the edge of a cliff, you hang on.

When you cope, you are attempting to address the undeniable changes you're experiencing while minimizing your distress. There are as many ways of coping with stress as there are people who face it. How we choose to navigate the ever-shifting terrain of our lives has a lot to do with both our orientation to life and the way we have handled challenges in the past. Janie Brown, a psychotherapist who works with cancer survivors, explains: "In my 20 years of experience, I have come to understand that most people revert back to previous patterns of behavior, which are complementary with their basic personality. So if they were optimistic and always saw difficulties as a glass half full, they will likely revert to optimism. And if they tended to be more negative, pessimistic or see the glass as half empty, they will likely approach their recovery in the same way." (6)

One coping mechanism common to cancer survivors is denial. To deny something is to declare it untrue or non-existent. Perhaps that is why denial is often our first reaction to painful news: *This can't be true!* Denial allows us to back gently into the grieving process, to pace ourselves by acknowledging and then adjusting slowly to our grief and loss. But although denial can be useful in the short term, over time it will not help you to address your ongoing recovery needs. It's as if you are reaching out to life with a closed fist rather than an open hand, clinging tightly to the old instead of being receptive to something new. It is only when you confront your struggles and begin to understand them that you'll be able to work out solutions. Acceptance facilitates a movement from coping to adapting, allowing you to develop strategies that will truly assist you in living well over time.

MOVING FORWARD

Any significant change in your life places you in situations where you are uncertain of how to act. With uncertainty comes discomfort. Before you can feel comfortable again, you must learn to do new things, or to do the same things in different ways. The transition from who you are to who you can become is dependent upon a willingness to let go, to learn to adapt. You will be leaving behind what is known and moving on towards the unknown.

While some ways of coping are useful as short-term responses to a crisis, they do not serve as adaptive strategies that work over time. Adaptation is crucial for effectively dealing with change. When we adapt, we modify and make adjustments, which helps us to face life's challenges head-on. Our ability to be flexible is based upon our ability to adapt, and it is flexibility that helps us to develop resilience.

Resilience is the capacity to bounce back, to recover from a temporary collapse and return to normal functioning. We draw upon our inner resilience to uncover new strength. With resilience, we learn to focus on the problems at hand and find ways to solve them. Resilience allows us to align those parts of ourselves that have changed with the parts that have remained the same.

Reorientation is another essential aspect of the second transition. Scars heal. You find new support in unexpected places. New questions arise. Reorientation is the process of continual self-appraisal. It involves re-establishing yourself in relation to your new circumstances, which may well require you to change direction or reinvent yourself. It may even require you to move backwards — unravelling — in order to get on with living the life you want.

During cancer's second transition, you will find yourself shifting from day-to-day coping to developing and experimenting with adaptive strategies for living well with the side effects of your cancer.

No single, magic strategy for adapting exists. Effective adapting may require acceptance and humour one day, confrontation the next. At times, you'll want to pursue your goals, but occasionally you may choose to do nothing. There is no right or wrong way to change. Becoming your own authority on what's right for your body, your health, and your life will take time, and it will require you to pay attention to what works for you.

WHAT SURVIVORS WANT

After treatment ends, many survivors are left on their own to discover new ways of coping. They need to develop successful adaptive strategies, and this is often done through trial and error. Although the road to healing is unique for everyone, survivors share common ground in the things they want after treatment. We've divided these wants into three categories:

- Idealistic wants
- Achievable wants
- Ultimate wants

Idealistic Wants

All survivors express three idealistic wants, regardless of the severity of their cancer or the intensity of their treatment:

- A guarantee that the cancer is gone and won't come back
- Reassurance that they are doing the right things to keep the cancer away
- A definite deadline by which they will feel normal again

Idealistic wants are by their nature unrealistic, though this does not diminish their strength or importance in your life. It is important to acknowledge these desires, but also to recognize that they are unattainable.

"My wife really wanted to have a baby. But first I needed a guarantee that I would be around for a while. I was very insecure, apprehensive, and anxious about how long I would be alive. I didn't think it was fair to introduce someone new to the world if I wasn't going to be here to help look after them."

— Roger, 32 years old, testicular cancer, 2-year survivor

Cancer treatment does not come with a worry-free, money-back guarantee. There will always be some people who do all the right things and still get sick or die, while others recover for no apparent reason. Rest, exercise, diet, medicine, prayer, and positive coping skills all have a beneficial impact on health. But there is no way to be sure that these activities will keep cancer away.

"I became a strict vegan and focused on eating foods rich in antioxidants. I continue to see my traditional Chinese medicine practitioner, and regularly practice relaxation with music to keep my stress levels low. I'm constantly reading about the body and how it works. But I just can't seem to get enough information. I often wonder — am I doing enough? Am I doing it right?"

— Theresa, 22 years old, melanoma, 1-year survivor

How long will it take to feel normal again? When will the fatigue end? When will you wake up and not think about cancer? Everyone is unique, and each survivor will recover differently. People long for and often request a specific time frame for their recovery phase, but even when one is given, it is often wrong. There is no infallible authority, no proven healing path that works for everyone. These questions do not have simple answers. What you face after treatment is the beginning of a process that involves figuring out the full effect cancer has had on you.

Achievable Wants

In order to move forward after treatment, you will need to decide how you want to live the rest of your life. Achievable wants are realistic, specific goals that help ease the transition from being a patient to living well. Survivors identify six of them:

- Guidelines
- Validation
- Support
- Empowerment
- Permission
- Reordered priorities

Guidelines. Survivors want a bridge or structured process to take them from treatment to full recovery. They want practical suggestions for taming their fears and anxieties, for alleviating stress, and for managing the various side effects of treatment.

> *"For several months after my treatments were finished, I continued to feel sick. My body was changing and my priorities were shifting dramatically. I longed for some kind of map or path to show me the way forward, something tangible to guide me through this uncomfortable experience."*
> — Drew, 46 years old, brain cancer, 18-month survivor

Validation. Survivors want to know that their fears and anxieties are normal. They have just gone through a traumatic, life-threatening event, and they want acknowledgment and understanding of the difficulties they have experienced.

> *"Sometimes people just don't realize I've been through hell, and although I'm on the other side of all the treatments, I'm still scared. They don't understand how hard it is to be back at work still so exhausted. They say things like, 'You must be so happy' or 'You're so lucky.' Sure I'm glad I'm alive, but how am I lucky? I'm lucky to have to live the rest of my life with a colostomy bag? I don't feel lucky."*
> — George, 41 years old, colon cancer, 9-week survivor

Support. Survivors want help sorting through their concerns and questions. They want someone with an open mind and a listening ear who will encourage them to become active participants in their own recovery.

> *"The feeling of leaving on the last day of radiation was overwhelming: 'What's next?' I would have liked somebody to take me under their wing and help me through this next phase. I was just as afraid as when I'd been diagnosed. I was on my own and going back to a life that was nothing like it had been before."*
> — Laurie, 32 years old, throat cancer, 5-month survivor

Permission. The types of permission that survivors seek are numerous and diverse. Some people want permission to say "no" to unwelcome burdens, jobs, or the demands of others. Some want permission to say "yes" to change. They want permission to explore new possibilities in their lives or to take the time they really need to heal.

> *"People's expectations aren't going to change, and they won't readily give me permission to change. I finally realized I needed to give myself permission to live my life the way I wanted."*
> — Kylie, 57 years old, uterine cancer, 7-year survivor

Empowerment. Empowerment means becoming your own authority on your body and your health. Survivors want to feel that they are captains of their own ships. They want to be able to take action on what's right for them, and to initiate changes that promote recovery and ongoing health.

> *"Throughout my cancer treatment, everyone had advice for me: stress management, anger management, time management. I didn't know what to do first. Finally I realized I was the only one who could decide what was right for me."*
> — Kathy, 44 years old, colon cancer, 1-year survivor

Reordered priorities. Many survivors want to make life changes that reflect the insights they have gained from their experience. They seek help in creating a new vision of the future in order to redefine their priorities and set new goals.

> *"Where do I start? What do I put at the top of my list? I don't know how much time I have left, but I want to make every day count."*
> — Jacques, 55 years old, prostate cancer, 2-month survivor

Ultimate Wants

Ultimate wants are more general in nature than idealistic or achievable wants, and perhaps harder to pin down, but they will set the tone for the rest of your life. Survivors share these wants with anyone moving through a major life transition, and fulfilling them may be a lifelong process.

- The ability to face mortality
- Inner peace
- An integration of old and new selves

The ability to face mortality. After a diagnosis of cancer, death is no longer merely theoretical. It may happen sooner than you had hoped or expected. Survivors want a way to make peace with the reality of death.

> *"Although I feel as if I've dodged a bullet, I know I'm not out of danger. I am more aware of the presence and possibility of death now, but I'm still afraid to die."*
> — Eric, 63 years old, colon cancer, 4-month survivor

Inner peace. Inner peace is a state of being that includes a calm mind, an open heart and a feeling of being centred. It involves letting go of how things used to be. To be at peace is to find that fine balance in life where you can identify problems, meet challenges head-on, do whatever the situation requires, then take a deep breath and allow the dust to settle.

"When I'm centred, I can keep perspective, see possibilities, and make wise choices. My challenge is to find that centre when I'm feeling overwhelmed with loss or fear."
                    — Loretta, 35 years old, leukemia, 3-year survivor

Integration. Integration involves reassembling the multiple pieces of your self into a unified whole. To be integrated means to address not only the physical and emotional effects of your cancer, but also the impact of the illness on your relationships and your spirituality. Integration ultimately brings contentment, wisdom and a feeling of being grounded in your life.

"I learned to take control of the things I can and not fear what I can't. My cancer experience has shown me an inner strength I didn't know I had."
                    — Pamela, 50 years old, ovarian cancer, 6-year survivor

Whether resuming life with renewed gusto or choosing to begin a new way of living, many survivors express the desire to live more authentically, in better alignment with their values, hopes, and dreams. They want to make new choices with confidence, to find peace, and to use the strength they've developed from cancer to guide them in the future. For many, new concerns arise that are closely linked with spirituality or a growing sense of greater connection with others and with the world.

START WHERE YOU ARE

Transforming your life is a thrilling prospect, but also a daunting one. If the caterpillar were given a choice, it would probably never undergo the frightening metamorphosis required to become a butterfly. Just how is this metamorphosis to be achieved for the cancer survivor? *Start where you are.* It sounds simple, but acknowledging and respecting your present physical and emotional state of health, as well as the health of your relationships and your spirit, are the foundational steps you must take in order to begin moving forward.

Progress will not happen overnight. Just like the rise and fall of the tides, all things happen according to their own rhythm. Changes that last take time and cannot be hurried. As much as we may long for spring in the midst of winter, it comes when the time is right.

All of us face the fear and frustration, even the suffering, that comes from not being able to stop the relentless waves of time and change. Often, just when we think we have it all under control, we suffer a setback and are reminded of how powerless we are. Despite our wish that life will hold firm, it never does. Life is a kaleidoscope — the slightest change will alter all the patterns.

It might help to remember that although not all changes are ones we can choose, change is an inevitable component of life. Seeing yourself as part of a continuum of perpetual change ultimately leads toward greater awareness and peace. You might even welcome change when you realize that old habits do not have to weigh down your new life. Your past doesn't have to become your future.

During cancer's second transition, your life will probably feel as fragmented as a complex jigsaw puzzle. What you are aiming for is to put these pieces together in order to move forward and feel whole or normal again. We've begun laying out some of the pieces of the puzzle. Let's look further at how the picture unfolds.

CHAPTER THREE

Laying Out the Pieces

"People often talk about the physical changes, but it's more than just what happens to your body. You find out a lot about yourself. First off, you realize you're very strong because you've survived some pretty terrible stuff you never thought you'd have to endure. Secondly, you sort through who and what is really important to you and you begin to live your life accordingly."

— Petra, 44 years old, leukemia, 4-month survivor

"My feelings didn't make sense. The crisis was over, and everything had turned out better than I had hoped. Why didn't I feel good? What was wrong with me?"

— Kathleen, 62 years old, breast cancer, 1-month survivor

A store-bought jigsaw puzzle comes with a picture on the box to show you what you'll be creating. For survivors, the larger picture becomes clear only when the puzzle is complete. In this chapter, we will describe how you can begin to move from surviving to living well. Using our four-phase process, you will take an active role in your health by choosing and designing your own Healing Plan. Through this process, you will assemble a new picture of yourself.

During recovery, you will confront the physical, social, emotional and spiritual consequences of cancer; they are a few of the pieces of the puzzle.

Assembling a puzzle usually isn't easy. The big picture doesn't always come together quickly. Some people will readily find the pieces they need, fit them together and move on. Others will find the process more of a challenge. The puzzle may sit on their coffee tables for weeks and months, maybe even years, as they come to the table, fit a few more pieces in, and then leave it alone. Finishing the puzzle of your recovery will require time, persistence and courage. You have to be ready to examine certain pieces closely, ask questions, and think carefully about how you will proceed. How you choose to solve this particular puzzle will affect the quality of your life both now and in the future.

Once you begin this task, you will notice certain puzzle shapes becoming familiar: curing, healing, and recovery. Perhaps the best way to start is to find out what these pieces mean.

CURING

The treatment plan developed for you by your health care team had a curative intent; they chose it with the expectation that it would eliminate the cancer and cure you. The word "cure" is usually used to describe a medical procedure that aims to eliminate disease or alleviate pain. When you undergo surgery, chemotherapy or radiation for cancer, you seek to be cured. Yet it is a rare doctor who tells a patient at the end of cancer treatment that he or she is cured. Instead, you're told you are in remission. What might that sound like to your ears? On hold. In limbo. Unable to proceed with the rest of your life until you have something more definite to hold onto.

HEALING

The word "heal" comes from the Old English "haelen," which means "to make whole." Healing is directed at restoring the body to health, homeostasis (equilibrium) or balance. While cure-oriented treatment originates from outside the person, healing is generated from within. Healing optimizes physical recovery and greatly enhances our quality of life. It integrates all aspects of our fragmented selves. We seek to heal and sustain ourselves when we participate in activities that challenge our bodies, engage our minds, and awaken our spirits. For example, we actively pursue healing when we eat a balanced diet, exercise regularly, indulge our creative passions, or delight in beautiful music.

In his book *Choices in Healing*, Michael Lerner writes, "Although healing and curing are different, they are entwined. For any cure to work, the physical healing power of the individual must be sufficient to enable recovery to take place. But healing goes beyond curing and may take place when curing is not at issue or has proved impossible. Although the capacity to heal physically is necessary to any successful cure, healing can also take place on deeper levels whether or not physical recovery occurs." (1)

Healing includes mending your physical wounds, recovering from emotional distress, and deepening your connections with loved ones, nature, and sometimes your God or Creator. It has the potential to unite mind, body, heart, and soul. Many of us conform to the expectations of others rather than living according to our own values, hopes and aspirations. By reclaiming a connection to your true self, you become actively engaged in the process of healing.

The healing process involves change, loss, resistance, and ultimately acceptance. For some people it ignites curiosity: *What else is there? Have I been missing something?* For others, it opens the door to full exploration, admitting hidden or forgotten dreams of becoming an artist, a writer, a violist, a scientist or an architect. Moving forward with the rest of your life, even though you are in remission from cancer, is not only possible, it is essential. But how do you get from here to there?

RECOVERY

When people talk about recovery, they often mean the process of restoring something to its normal condition — though by now the word normal should ring alarm bells for you. But there is another way to look at recovery, and that is as reclaiming something that has been lost. The most obvious thing you lose when you have cancer is your health. Yet, in speaking to survivors, we have discovered that recovery from cancer involves more than just regaining your physical balance. It's a question of establishing a new centre of gravity.

Recovery is not so much about moving on as it is about moving through change. That's why each person's experience will be different. Your recovery will be affected by many factors, including the number of changes you've experienced, the degree of those changes, your ability to cope, and your capacity to adapt and work with change.

The process of recovery encompasses four distinct components:

- Recovering a sense of self
- Recovering a sense of control
- Recovering a sense of meaning
- Recovering a sense of future

THE FOUR-PHASE PROCESS OF RECOVERY

In Chapter Two we showed you how cancer creates two back-to-back transitions and said that we would focus on the second transition, from surviving to living well. Our four-phase recovery process will assist you on your way.

The four-phase process of recovery will help you put together the puzzle of your life after cancer. First, you will find the four corners (the Inquiry Phase). Next, you will frame in the edges (the Discovery Phase). From there, you'll work towards the centre (the Growth Phase), and finally you'll come to see the whole picture (the Reflection Phase). Each one of the phases is just as important as the others.

From diagnosis through treatment, every cancer experience is unique. So, too, is each person's path to recovery. Consequently, although we provide the structure for recovery, you will constantly be tailoring it to suit your needs. That is why the process will work for you as it has for numerous other cancer survivors: it will be your own.

1. The Inquiry Phase — Recovering a Sense of Self

Cancer is a frightening and life-changing experience. No one who lives through its diagnosis and treatment will come out unscathed. Cancer can disrupt your career, alter your appearance, and change your relationships. It can distort the picture you have of your current life and skew your hopes and dreams for the future. At the heart of the cancer experience is a shift in identity that can be not just confusing but completely disorienting. *Who am I now?* many survivors find themselves asking. In his book *It's Not about the Bike*, Lance Armstrong describes the effect being diagnosed with the disease had on him: "Cancer would change everything for me. It wouldn't just derail my career; it would deprive me of my entire definition of who I was." (2)

The goal of the Inquiry Phase is to help you recover your sense of self. This phase is the time to take stock of the impact cancer has had on you. You'll be on a fact-finding mission, conducting a personal inventory to figure out who you are post-treatment. Critical to this phase is the need to acknowledge the physical, emotional, social and spiritual changes you've experienced because of the cancer and its treatments, regardless of whether these changes are subtle or involve a 180-degree shift in how you live your life.

Key questions you'll be asking yourself during the Inquiry Phase include the following:

- In what ways have I remained the same, and in what ways have I become someone new?
- What have I gained and what have I lost through my cancer experience?
- How do I pick up some of the pieces of my life and leave others behind?

The essential first step in assembling a complex jigsaw puzzle is to find the four corners. In the Inquiry Phase, we introduce the Self-Scan, which will provide you with a structured method for assessing the four corners of your experience with cancer: how it has affected your body, your emotions, your spirit and your relationships.

While we expect to grieve the loss of a loved one, we are unprepared for — even shocked by — the magnitude of loss that comes with a life-threatening illness. Cancer's losses can take many forms. The most evident of these is physical. But you may also have experienced a loss of income or savings, the loss of your job, the loss of important relationships or favourite pastimes. You may be struggling too with the more elusive loss of trust in your own body, your ability to control your life, and your faith in the future. Along with determining what has changed in your life, you will also take the time during the Inquiry Phase to grieve the losses — large and small, tangible and intangible — that have occurred due to cancer and its treatments.

2. The Discovery Phase — Recovering a Sense of Control

While you are in treatment for cancer, many things are outside your control. Although we can never fully control what happens in our lives, a diagnosis of cancer can leave you feeling fearful and powerless, unable to move forward. The goal of the Discovery Phase is to help you recover a sense of control. Beginning with small, manageable choices, you will learn to take charge of your life once again. You can't control cancer, but you can empower yourself by taking action based on new perspectives.

During this phase, the following key questions will arise:

- How can I become an active participant in my recovery?
- What is possible in my life?
- Am I living the life I want to live?
- What is my vision of living well?

When you are tired and in pain, it can seem overwhelming to face such enormous and difficult questions. During the Discovery Phase, we will help you identify what drains your energy and what replenishes it. Creating the life you want takes courage and determination. No one else knows what you are experiencing. That's why it's important that you acknowledge your own need to heal and then give yourself permission to proceed with your own recovery, whether that means taking six months off work or joining a support group while maintaining your daily routine. In this phase of recovery, you'll develop a Healing Plan and craft a Vision Statement to help you explore your needs and desires.

In his book *The Hero with a Thousand Faces,* Joseph Campbell presents a composite picture of the heroic quest that individuals embark upon when they step forward to live a more integrated, authentic life. Old ideals and emotional patterns may no longer fit. Campbell's call to adventure echoes cancer's wake-up call: it is time to now take charge of your life and your destiny. (3)

In the Inquiry Phase, you set out the four corners of the recovery puzzle. As you work through the Discovery Phase, you will be framing in the edges and learning to give your life a tangible structure.

3. The Growth Phase — Recovering a Sense of Meaning

The Growth Phase of recovery involves working towards the puzzle's centre, where meaning lies. Many survivors express the need to make sense of their cancer experience, to understand it and put it into context so that they can move on with their lives.

It is not uncommon for people who have come through a life-threatening trauma to say that they really didn't appreciate the peaks in their lives until they had experienced the valleys. Harvesting the positive insights from your cancer experience is not an easy process. But ultimately, it will allow you to reassess your life. During the Growth Phase, you will utilize your strengths and supports to develop strategies for moving toward your vision of living well. The key questions that emerge during this phase will include:

- What new insights have I gleaned from this experience? In what ways have they made me stronger?
- How have my priorities changed?
- What new clarity does my life now have?

Cancer can be the wake-up call to a renewed purpose in life or to getting your life back on track. Many survivors describe it as a turning point, the catalyst that propels them to make changes they never dreamed possible. Cancer shakes your illusions of immortality. It robs you of the sense of invincibility and innocence that once protected you. But what replaces that feeling is infinitely more valuable: a new awareness and a mature understanding of both life and death.

At this point in the puzzle, you will find the bigger picture starting to take shape. When you know what you want from life, it gives you both hope and direction. Recovering a sense of meaning will give you the courage you need to move forward.

4. The Reflection Phase — Recovering a Sense of the Future

While none of us knows how much time we have ahead, this awareness is heightened for the cancer survivor. During treatment, your immediate situation is challenge enough. In the back of your mind there is always the possibility that you won't have a future to worry about. But after the treatments finish, your anxieties and fears about that uncertain future — if left unchecked — can interfere with your enjoyment of life's simple pleasures and your ability to live in the present moment.

The goal of the Reflection Phase is to help you recover a sense of the future. This is the time to step back, take a deep breath and consider the puzzle you have assembled. While you must learn to live with the uncertainty of tomorrow, it is also integral to your recovery to plan for your future.

During the Reflection Phase, new questions will arise:

- How do I learn to accept uncertainty and live with the fear of recurrence?
- How do I integrate change into my life?
- How do I live for today and plan for tomorrow?
- What is next for me?

The Reflection Phase is a time of quiet contemplation. Because our society is so focused on doing and accomplishing, it is a challenge to find such time. It is even more of a challenge to allow yourself to take it. But it is critically important that you do so. Your ultimate goal during the Reflection Phase will be to cultivate a sense of inner peace. It is not until you come to terms with your struggles with cancer, acknowledge your pain and suffering and then let it settle, that you can move forward into the future.

NO TIME LIMIT

Because you will tailor this four-phase process to suit your own life and recovery needs, there is no specific time frame for it. Some parts of the process will take longer to complete than others. Yet to successfully navigate this transition, you must address the key themes in all four phases. It takes time to really acknowledge and grieve your losses, to truly explore possibilities, and to find meaning in a major life-changing event.

Recovery happens one day at a time. Accompanying you on your daily quest will be two essential practices: attentive walking and the five-question check-in. These practices will complement the process we've described in this chapter and help you take active steps every day towards living well.

It's time to take a closer look at these practices and take those first steps right now.

CHAPTER FOUR

The Daily Practices

"Cancer asks so much of you. It asks you to review your life and your relationship to your body, mind, and spirit; it asks you to reconsider your beliefs and attitudes and goals. I started to explore the possibilities presenting themselves in my life, to really ask myself what my choices were, and most importantly, if they were healthy ones."

— Jolene, 49 years old, ovarian cancer, 5-month survivor

"I felt like I had been living according to some prewritten script, playing a role in the production of my life. Now I understand that the drama called 'my life' requires me to perform live, rewriting every second as it goes on."

— Leanne, 33 years old, melanoma, 3-year survivor

We believe a simple, consistent daily practice that integrates body, mind, heart and spirit is an essential first step to recovering a sense of wholeness. Why? By creating a habit of turning inward and paying attention to your thoughts and feelings, you'll become more attuned to those quiet yearnings. You'll learn how to notice changes, listen to what's being revealed, and trust your new voice. You'll become more aware of the various aspects of yourself and how you interact with your surroundings.

The American College Dictionary describes practice as "a repeated or habitual performance for the purpose of acquiring skill or proficiency." (1) As a child, you were probably told that you had to practice in order to achieve your goals, whether that meant learning to play a musical instrument or becoming an athlete. Consequently, you may believe that practice is merely a means to an end, useful only for the results it brings. But some types of practice are valuable for the process itself.

As you move from being a survivor to living well with cancer, you are turning immediate coping skills into long-term adaptive strategies. In order to do this, you will probably have to learn some new habits that support healthy choices. Daily practice not only fosters the development of new habits but encourages the reflective time that is so critical to a sense of perspective.

Psychologists tell us that it takes at least three weeks of steady, determined repetition for a new behaviour to become habitual. But we live in chaotic, distracting and demanding times. The most insidious enemy of a daily practice is our North American culture's relentless celebration of immediate gratification. The quick fix is evident in fast weight-loss diets, thrill-a-minute movies, and "how to do anything in one minute" books. Amid such a din, it is difficult to be patient and to commit to the more distant, yet enduring, changes that come from a regular, long-lasting practice.

The two practices we have designed are practical, straightforward and accessible: attentive walking and the five-question check-in. Once you make the decision to try them, it's important to acknowledge these practices as worthwhile activities that you undertake on a regular basis. These are the first steps towards giving yourself permission to take control of your own health. When you participate in the daily practices, you are truly taking care of yourself.

Daily practice is a time to mine your own life experiences and digest the events of your healing journey. Both of the practices we've developed involve acknowledging and accepting change — core elements in the recovery process. Do them, and we guarantee you will see results over time.

1. ATTENTIVE WALKING

We are all part of a larger world that extends past our front door into our communities and beyond. Regular, repetitive exercise that takes you out into your surroundings is both soothing and stimulating. As you stretch your legs and open your heart and mind to the world around you, you are also entering the recovery process.

Walking is the simplest, cheapest and most convenient form of exercise. Newspapers and magazines regularly carry articles extolling its merits. A walk is not only good for your heart, muscles, and lungs. It can also reduce anxiety and quiet your fears.

A daily practice of attentive walking combines physical exercise with sensory input and personal awareness. It will help you regain a foothold in your life. Attentive walking will:

- activate and strengthen your physical body
- release and calm your mind
- engage your spirit
- enhance your relationship with yourself

The daily practice of attentive walking is just that — daily! We recommend 20 minutes, depending on your fatigue level. Start where you can. If you can only walk for two or three minutes, begin there, and build up to your 20 minutes of continuous walking gradually.

How do you do attentive walking? It couldn't be easier. Anywhere, at any time of day, go out for a walk. This is not a sweat-drenched hike that demands immense effort, nor is it a frenzied race-walk designed to cover the most ground possible. Your only goal is to be fully aware of both your body and your surroundings, to experience the moment.

Your daily walk is a time to get reacquainted with your body, to notice and feel yourself moving through space, to find joy in physical activity. Don't think of it as exercise; think of it as movement. Feel your feet making con-tact with the ground. Pay attention to how your arms move through the air. Tune in to the shifts and bends and forward motion of your hips and legs.

Listen to your body's signals as you walk, too. Do you feel tired? Energized? Are you calm and quiet, or frantic and hurried? Do you feel sick to your stomach? Does your arm ache?

Pay attention to your breath as well. Notice that when you inhale your chest rises, and when you exhale your chest lowers and falls inward. Is your inhalation longer or shorter than your exhalation? Are you breathing deeply from your belly, or is your breath shallow and quick, from the chest area only?

Is your breathing tight, deep, heavy? Are you huffing and puffing?

What about your stride? Do your arms swing freely? Do you land hard on your heels? Does your right foot feel the same as your left?

Focusing on your body will probably sound simple until you go for your first attentive walk. Then, instead of blissfully reflecting upon your breathing, you may find yourself thinking that the car needs new brakes or remembering that your son needs to be picked up from soccer practice, and what will you make for dinner tonight, anyhow? Your inner worrier has found a captive audience.

Sometimes we go for a walk to work things out, but that is not the purpose of attentive walking. In your daily practice you are not on a mission to solve anything, but instead to allow life to unfold in front of you. While it is normal for everyday concerns to intrude upon your 20 minutes of peace, resist the temptation to let them take over. Acknowledge them, and then let them go. The idea is always to return to the present moment.

The purpose of attentive walking is to encourage you to reconnect with your body. In our busy lives, many of us habitually function from the neck up. Reorienting yourself towards your body will require you to listen to its needs and then trust in the wisdom of what it's telling you. Do you respond when your body gives you early warning signals through pain or fatigue, telling you to slow down? Or do you ignore these signals and push ahead, only to suffer the consequences later?

Our intention with the practice of attentive walking is to create a peaceful oasis in your day where you are paying attention to the person you are now. That's why we encourage you to walk alone and in silence, so that you can truly consider what is happening both within and around you. Attentive walking places equal emphasis on your body, mind, and spirit. As you quiet your mind and connect to the spirit within, attentive walking will lead you to increased clarity, self-awareness and strength.

We recommend that you take time to notice not only your movements, but also the smells, sights, and sounds around you. Who and what do you perceive? Maybe it's the smell of bacon frying at the local café. Maybe it's the exhaust fumes from the car idling at the red light. Notice the glitter of fresh snow, or how green the leaves are, or how the hairs stand up on a squirrel's tail.

Focus on details. If you usually walk past the red house on the corner, pay attention to the patterns on the lawn, the textures, the shades of red, the weathered wood panel around the door. Notice how the people around you walk quickly during the week but seem to relax their pace on the weekend. Notice differences in temperature and wind direction and feel the warmth of the sun upon your face. Take in the colours and sounds around you, instead of rushing past them. Remember, it's not the destination that's important; it's each step, each movement, each breath. Be attentive and aware, and don't worry about counting the laps.

As often as you can, walk outside, since variations in the weather will affect your experience. Even the most determined walker can be discouraged by intense heat or ice underfoot, but don't let the weather break your habit. Find a shopping mall or an indoor track for those days when outdoor walking proves impossible.

You can even make attentive walking practical. Do it in the time it takes you to walk to the bus on your way to work. Go on your lunch break, or take a longer route back to your car. The point of this practice is to teach you to slow down, pay attention and be fully present. When or where you do it is less important than your commitment to doing it daily.

Attentive Walking: Summary
- Set aside 20 minutes to walk alone every day.
- Pay attention to your breath.
- Notice what's happening in your body. What's your stride like? Do you move freely and easily? Where do you feel pain, tightness, or discomfort?
- Pay attention to sounds, colours, and smells as you walk.
- Notice the feelings that come up as you give your attention to the world around you.
- Come back to the present moment whenever your mind wanders off.

2. THE FIVE-QUESTION CHECK-IN
The second component of your daily practice is the five-question check-in. This is a brief interval — just five minutes daily — during which you take stock of your day and record your thoughts and feelings in a recovery journal.

While it may be clear immediately how attentive walking will assist your ongoing recovery, the benefits of the check-in will become more apparent over time. Completing the check-in may stimulate, irritate, or surprise you, but doing it regularly will help you to clarify the choices and changes you need to make in order to live the life you want.

Each of the five questions in the check-in requires you to think about a certain aspect of yourself. This ensures that none of the components of your life is ignored or pushed aside. It's easy to lose track of one aspect of yourself when other areas dominate. Some days, certain questions may be easy to answer; other days, you might feel challenged by all of them. But each plays an important part in your recovery process.

These are the five questions you'll be asking yourself daily:

1. What's happening with my body?
2. How am I feeling emotionally?
3. When I let my thoughts wander, what do I find myself thinking about?
4. Who did I connect with today?
5. What gave me a sense of peace?

There are no right or wrong answers to any of these questions. This practice doesn't require any exceptional skills or special thinking. It takes only a few minutes of your time, yet this check-in will provide you with remarkable information as you become your own observer and recorder of day-to-day changes. Nothing is too petty or inconsequential to record. Over time, you will recognize patterns and find yourself generating new thoughts and ideas about your health and recovery.

"I couldn't believe it. I thought I was afraid most days. But after three weeks of recording the answers to my check-in, I noticed a change. My thoughts and feelings were moving from fear to gratitude. I was becoming more aware of what was going on around me and appreciating simple things like the sounds of the children playing in the backyard next door."
— Ivan, 51 years old, prostate cancer, 2-month survivor

"It's hard to think about your heart's longings when you're in pain or exhausted or dealing with side effects such as lymphedema or hot flashes. But because of the daily check-in questions, I began to notice other aspects of my life. I thought more about where I was finding a sense of peace and who filled me with joy and who didn't. I became more aware of my wants and needs than I had in years."

— Tamara, 37 years old, breast cancer, 3-year survivor

Here's an example of how your check-in might look on a particular day:

1. **What's happening with my body?** My shoulder is stiff and I have a headache. I'm tired but was happy to be able to get to the grocery store. My back pain is getting better. I had lunch with Sue and was able to sit comfortably the entire time.

2. **How am I feeling emotionally?** I'm angry at my sister, Jeanie, for treating me like an invalid. I'm sad and often scared of the future. I felt moments of intense joy while walking through the park today.

3. **When I let my thoughts wander, what do I find myself thinking about?** I need to let others know that I can't take on any more tasks at work. I'm concerned about my health benefits, as well as about how I'm going to pay my mortgage. I think about making amends with my brother; we haven't spoken since his birthday four years ago.

4. **Who did I connect with today?** Dad called and we talked for ten minutes. I felt a strong connection with God when I went out into the garden.

5. **What gave me a sense of peace?** Sitting alone on the patio with my coffee and my dog in my lap. The half-hour I spent reading Toni Morrison's new book.

Consider where in your home you will go to reflect and record your responses to these questions every day. Some survivors designate a certain chair or set up a special space where they can be alone with their thoughts. You'll need both silence and breathing room to ponder these questions. Only then will you be able to hear your inner voice.

Consider, too, what form your recovery journal will take. It doesn't matter whether you write by hand in a fancy journal or spiral notebook or create a file on your computer. The important thing is that you have a safe, comfortable place to record your thoughts each day. Your recovery journal is where you will write your truth from that raw place in your heart. Be honest in your responses. What you write is for your eyes only. Your recovery journal will become your change-tracking system, progress map, and diary all in one. As you monitor your thoughts and feelings, you will see yourself moving from fragmentation towards wholeness.

In setting up your journal, we suggest you first copy the five check-in questions in a place where you can refer to them easily. Then, for each day's entry, write the date at the top of the page and leave enough space for your answers.

DATE: MARCH 16, 2006
Five-Question Check-In

1.

2.

3.

4.

5.

Once you have begun the practice of the five-question check-in, you may find insights or glimmers of inspiration coming to you at other times of the day — on your way to work, for example, or while preparing supper. Some survivors carry a small notepad with them to jot down thoughts they can include in their daily check-in later on.

Five-Question Check-In: Summary

- Create a time and space at the end of each day where you can be alone with your thoughts.
- Sit for a moment in silence and take a few deep breaths.
- Ask yourself each question and listen attentively to what you think and feel.
- Write short answers to each question. Don't deliberate or worry about spelling or grammar; just record what comes to mind.
- Be honest with yourself. Remember, no one will read this except you.

MAKING THE PRACTICES WORK

Why do some survivors stick with daily exercises and develop healthy habits, while others give up? When it comes to motivation, we're all unique. That means you will need to find out what motivates you most effectively. This is the time to ask yourself what kind of role you want to take in your own recovery.

Nutritionist Kathleen Fell works with cancer survivors on their diet and eating habits: "I spend a lot of time talking with my clients about their will to live. I ask them, 'How much effort are you willing to put into your health and wellness? Are you prepared to take time for self-care?' Their answers affect whether or not they end up making good meals three times a day or not. What a person chooses to do for themselves may be an indication of their commitment to their health." (2)

Certainly, after cancer, fear is one of the strongest motivators for change. But while negative motivation can serve as the initial impetus for change, human nature is such that, over time, fear wanes and we return to old habits. That is why positive motivators such as the strong desire to look, feel, and be well are necessary for a long-term commitment to recovery and change.

You must be clear about your intentions: what exactly do you want to do with your life now that you've survived?

> *"I want to get better and live with more gusto. I want to give back. I have so much to live for and be grateful for. Once I started to focus on wellness instead of on the disease, I realized I was doing the right thing. I can take care of myself, eat well, meditate, exercise, and be less dependent on my wife for my daily care. I am on the road to recovery."*
> — Jack, 54 years old, lymphoma, 3-month survivor

Three crucial components will help make the daily practices work for you:

- Permission
- Attention
- Support

Permission

As a survivor of cancer, you have an opportunity to rethink your life, to choose to continue the things that contribute to your well-being and to abandon anything that does not. Giving yourself permission to actively work through your recovery requires a willingness to cooperate with change. It involves being eager to explore new possibilities, being open to the unknown, and being willing to reconsider your life with an open mind.

> *"I decided if I didn't give myself permission to heal now, when would I? So I told my family and friends I needed time to recover fully, and they all understood."*
> — Maureen, 46 years old, brain cancer, 2-year survivor

This is a time in your life when people will give you permission to make changes. But you're the one who must decide to use this time of transition as an investment in your ongoing healing. If you can do this, you will alter your relationship with the future.

Attention

We are socially and culturally trained to look outside ourselves for answers, but this is a time to train yourself to turn inward and listen. Becoming aware of the changes in your body means paying attention to what your body tells you. It takes discipline and commitment to pay attention. Although we may notice, and initially complain about, changes in our body, we quickly become accustomed to these and hardly perceive the corresponding changes we make to accommodate them. Your task is to build a new relationship with your body in order to see where and how it is changing.

Paying attention to the present moment also involves turning outward to the world around you, reawakening your senses to make yourself a close observer of life. You might try seeing yourself as a detective gathering clues about what is really going on in and around your life.

> *"When I consciously walk I notice the world more — the trees, the flowers, the clouds. But when I rush through my day, it all goes by me unnoticed. It seems you only become aware of what you actually make an effort to pay attention to."*
>
> — Bruce, 64 years old, lymphoma, 6-month survivor

Support

Now is the time to enlist the support of others. Be clear about what you want from your allies: encouragement, honesty, no judgment, feedback. Tell your husband, wife, mother, kids, whomever, that you are still healing and need time to work on your recovery. Let them know what you are doing and how they can help.

> *"I called my best friend, Joan, and said, 'I'm starting a new recovery program and I need your support. I want you to call me every few days and make sure I've done my walking and check-in exercise.' I'm committed to this process but I feel better knowing I've got a back-up in case I need it."*
>
> — Isabelle, 43 years old, lung cancer, 5-week survivor

There may also be occasions when you'll want to seek professional help as another way of taking charge of your health. Many survivors choose to visit a counsellor or join a support group to share their story with others. Don't forget: the most important ally you have is your core self. It is your beacon of strength, the light of hope that shines deep within you, guiding you forward. When times get hard, remind yourself of all you have been through, especially your past successes, and draw strength from that.

MAKING THE COMMITMENT

We have now laid out all the pieces you'll need to begin creating your recovery plan. Together, the two daily practices and the four-phase process we'll be describing in the rest of the book will help you rebuild the structure of your life — and assist you in finding your new normal. Only you can give yourself permission to make the commitment required to start this project.

This process belongs to you. You will develop a unique Healing Plan and Vision Statement that meet your own recovery needs. But you will not be alone. The voices of other survivors will guide and support you along the way.

Be gentle with yourself. You've come a long way already.

TOUCHING BASE

At the end of several chapters you will find what we call a Touching Base, it's our way of asking you how you're doing. Touching bases are meant predominantly as a form of encouragement and support for you as you do the two Daily Practices — Attentive Walking and the Five-Question Check-In. They offer further insights to some of the changes that may occur while you're participating in these two daily practices and they suggest ideas to enhance your recovery process. Look for them at the end of chapters six, nine, twelve and fifteen.

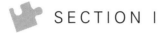 SECTION I

Finding the Four Corners: Inquiry

RECOVERING A SENSE OF SELF

The Self Scans

T he transition from surviving a life-threatening illness to living well is a time of sorting, assessing and regrouping. It is during this transition that you will strive to integrate your pre- and post-cancer selves. Some people use the metaphor of Humpty Dumpty: they have had a great fall and now need help to put themselves back together again. What is difficult to accept is that the reassembled pieces often don't fit back together in exactly the same way. During the recovery process, you will be grappling with some crucial questions: *How do I pick up some of the pieces of my life and let others go? How do I learn to accept this newly reconstructed me?*

There is no escaping the fact: recovery takes time. Your recovery will depend on the type of cancer you had, its severity, and the treatment you received, as well as your health before the diagnosis. Returning to everyday routines after a life-threatening illness is a big hurdle to leap. Many survivors find recovery even more emotionally taxing than their cancer treatment was. To make matters worse, having cancer does not make your other problems disappear (though it might eventually help put them in a different perspective). All the life issues you were struggling with before cancer will still be waiting for you once you walk out those hospital doors. Fatigue, chronic pain, and fear may even exacerbate them.

Remember the concept of the core self that we discussed in Chapter Two? That core self has seen you through this challenge. It has provided you with the strength and resilience you needed to survive. What you'll come to understand through the Inquiry Phase outlined in this section of the book is how that essential core keeps you stable as it moves you forward through ongoing change. It is your core self that helps you navigate transition and ultimately integrate old and new. As you observe the core at work and begin to trust it again, you will rebuild confidence in your choices and regain a sense of control.

No matter how much others may wish to help you, you must take charge of your own healing process. Only you really know what your current challenges are. Just because your wounds have closed or your hair has grown back, you are not necessarily healed. Healing is not about fixing; it's about responding to the changes you are faced with and learning to live with them.

WHAT IS A SELF SCAN?

The Inquiry process is a fact-finding mission, a way to take personal inventory to figure out what has changed in your life and what has remained the same. In order to cope with change, it is important to understand both your strengths and your limitations. Your biggest asset is self-knowledge. And don't let the word "limitations" scare you. Acknowledging weakness does not mean you are flawed; it means you are moving towards an acceptance of the changes cancer has brought into your life.

As you follow our program, you will conduct this personal inventory by using our four Self Scans. A Self Scan is a structured method of self-assessment that will help you identify the changes that have occurred because of the cancer and/or its treatments. Each Self Scans ask questions. You will provide the answers. In this way, you will establish a baseline from which to monitor the changes you've observed over time. From this baseline, you will create a Healing Plan that includes the strategies you need to move forward.

Let's return to our puzzle metaphor for a minute. Once the pieces of a jigsaw puzzle have been laid out, finding the four corners is the first step towards constructing the whole picture. Each of the following four chapters ends with a Self Scan that will help you identify areas of your life where cancer has caused significant changes or left side effects that are difficult to manage. The scans will also help you recognize your current strengths and abilities and identify the avenues of support available to you.

Recovery occurs in all aspects of the self. Our Self Scans give you the opportunity to assess yourself in four primary areas:

- **Body** — your physical abilities and skills
- **Mind** — your attitudes and beliefs
- **Spirit** — your sense of meaning and life's purpose
- **Relationships** — your social and family connections

Through this process of guided inquiry, you will take stock of what you know about your post-cancer self and also discover many things you may not have known before. We invite you on a journey of self-assessment as you begin your recovery process.

FINDING YOUR FOUR CORNERS: HOW TO DO THE SELF SCANS

For the sake of clarity, we have treated body, mind, spirit, and relationships as separate entities, although of course they are closely interconnected. Since cancer is a physical illness, we have chosen to start with the body, but that need not be where you begin. Perhaps it's your emotional turmoil that is shouting for attention, or maybe it's the needs of your spirit. For some people, relationship changes take priority. Each Self Scan represents a doorway to an aspect of yourself, a means of reviewing the most common side effects and issues pertaining to that area. Some of the survivorship issues we present will be more relevant to you than others. We suggest you begin in the area that interests you most. However, an important note: although it doesn't matter which scan you do first, you will need to work through all four of them before proceeding to the next phase of your recovery.

When you're assembling a puzzle, there are times you can't find the right piece no matter how hard you look. Life is like that too. We get stuck in thought patterns that keep us from seeing what's right in front of us. Often we get frustrated or discouraged. So a word of advice here: if you find yourself resisting a particular Self Scan, try moving to another corner of the puzzle.

You can return later to the one that was difficult.

As you read through the following four chapters, you'll see references to specific Self Scan questions. You can flip to the appropriate Self Scan and answer these questions as you go, or wait and complete the scan once you've read the entire chapter. How you approach the Self Scans will also depend to a certain extent on your energy level. Do as much as you can in one sitting, and then put the scan away. Return to it when you're ready, until eventually all four scans are complete. Most people find it takes between 30 minutes and an hour to complete a Self Scan, but there's no time limit, and it's definitely not a race. Take the time you need to answer the questions thoughtfully and honestly. Your answers will provide you with invaluable information.

As you progress through the Inquiry process, you will need to:

- **Find a quiet place** where you can concentrate and answer each Self Scan's thought-provoking questions. You can do the scan alone or with a partner. However, you may not feel comfortable talking about side effects such as incontinence or impotence with another person. If you do decide to go through the scan with a partner, choose someone you can be totally honest with, so that you won't be tempted to hide or alter the truth.

- **Write down your answers**. Writing your answers in your recovery journal (the same one you're using for your responses to the daily Five-Question Check-In) will help you to develop your Healing Plan. Later, your written responses will allow you to track your progress and review self-initiated changes.

- **Start where you are**. Whether you are two days out of treatment or two years, you'll want to start by assessing where you are today.

- **Trust in the process**. There are no right or wrong answers. The recovery process is about finding your own way. Acknowledge and respect the place you're in now. Trust in yourself and in the process to move you forward.

- **Honour your strengths and abilities.** Although you may feel compromised and vulnerable after your encounter with cancer, you actually have more strengths than limitations. It is hard to see this if you are focusing solely on loss, so it's important to honour the positive while you are assessing what has changed in your life.

- **Find support wherever you can.** Your family and friends may not realize that you need their support for ongoing recovery and healing. You might have to tell them. Surround yourself with people who are positive and encouraging. You don't need sympathy, but you will need compassion, and at times you may need to ask for help. Think about who in your life can stand by your side and help you get back on track as you move through this process.

- **Be brave.** It can be hard to look honestly at the changes that have occurred, rather than hiding from them, ignoring them, or minimizing them. Take a deep breath and acknowledge your current reality. Don't back away. You have survived and are moving forward, regardless of the difficulties.

- **Be patient and tender with yourself.** You are in recovery. Go slowly, and pay attention to what is happening both in and around you. Now is the time to step back, acknowledge and validate the journey you have taken.

SEEK THE MEDICAL HELP YOU NEED

While the four Self Scans offer an overview of many survivor issues and side effects, they do not represent an in-depth assessment for each type of cancer. They are only a framework, providing you with a helpful tool that you can use for yourself or as a basis for further conversations with your doctor and other members of your health care team, as well as with your family and friends.

We encourage you to seek the help you may need with your recovery. Your concerns, whatever they are, are valid. Don't hide them or feel that they're unworthy of your doctor's time. It's important to get the assistance you require, and no problem is too small to be addressed. You don't have to live with side effects, and you should not accept the view that they are a small price to pay for surviving cancer. If the health care professional you're seeing doesn't listen or take your concerns seriously, consider switching to someone who will.

> *"I felt sheepish about troubling my doctor with my problems; after all, I had just survived cancer. But eventually I asked for help, and she was surprised I hadn't told her about the side effects earlier. She helped me address each concern, and I started feeling better soon."*
> — Donna, 54 years old, ovarian cancer, 4-year survivor

Finally, remember that you are unique — your cancer experience is shaped by a multitude of factors related to the type of cancer you had, the treatment you received, your body chemistry, your personality, and so on. Because of this, you may experience changes that are very different from someone else's, even if they had the same type of cancer and received the same treatment. You are a complex person with needs, wants, hopes, and your own physical reality, all of which affect your emotional, social, spiritual and physical well-being. As you learn how to live with cancer, you will need to decipher, choose, create, and customize your goals to fit your life circumstances. The Self Scans are the all-important first step on this journey of recovery.

CHAPTER FIVE

In Your Skin: Assessing Your Body

"I felt like a broken tea cup. All of the pieces were lying on the floor and I knew I could glue them back together, but I also knew that the cup would be fragile and never quite the same again."

— Stephanie, 49 years old, lymphoma, 7-week survivor

"I'm left with a big scar on my back. I've lost confidence in how my body looks. I was at the beach recently for the first time since the surgery. Someone asked about the scar and I just didn't want to get into it, so I made up a story about a shark attack. They knew it wasn't true, but they let it go."

— Joe, 24 years old, lung cancer, 2-year survivor

If you were to walk into our office today, we would take a thorough history of your cancer experience and ask you questions about how you are feeling, how you function on a day-to-day basis, and which areas of your life you think need the most attention. What we would be giving you is, in effect, a starting line: a clear assessment of your needs and concerns, in order for you to begin the recovery process. That is our aim with these Self Scans. This chapter initiates the Inquiry process by exploring the impact that cancer and its treatments have had on your body.

Cancer jolts you back into your body. Physical symptoms and side effects force you to notice your physical self, often for the first time. The Self Scan at the end of this chapter will help you to become more curious about your body and to explore the ways in which it currently functions.

YOUR MOST PRECIOUS POSESSION

Many of us talk about our bodies as if we don't fully inhabit them. Because of our busy lives, we often live a short distance from our bodies, not always acknowledging the sensations and changes we experience day to day. Many survivors experience a definite dissociation from their physical bodies after cancer. Your task now is to rediscover your body and to learn to live with it and care for it again. Reclaiming your body and adapting to your new physical self are essential to the recovery process.

> "I think the hardest thing was learning how to walk again. That sounds very odd, but without breasts, your center of gravity shifts. I found the first few months after my surgery, I could easily lose my balance. I am still figuring out how to walk with good posture and comfortably, so that I am not tightening the muscles so much in my lower back or shoulders."
>
> — Judy, 53 years old, breast cancer, 1-year survivor

Recovering a sense of self within your body requires you to become fully aware of all five senses — listening in and surrendering to, rather than resisting, the day-to-day fluctuations in energy, symptoms and emotions that accompany healing. We encourage you to pay attention to what is happening to, in, and around your body right now. Become aware of its reactions. Remember, your body is your most precious possession. How you treat it is critical to your enjoyment of life.

SEEING FROM THE INSIDE OUT

We live in a culture that worships physical beauty and perfection. Cancer represents our worst fears of our bodies becoming less than whole, not measuring up to societal norms. There are an infinite number of body shapes, sizes and features, yet society tries to convince us that only a few of them are desirable. Before cancer you may have focused on your body's outward appearance, relating to yourself from the perspective of how you looked rather than how you felt. Now you'll be turning that perspective inside out and looking at your body differently.

Many cancer survivors tell us they feel bruised or broken, that cancer has left a big dent in their lives. The outward changes in your appearance may be obvious, such as scars, radiation burns, or the loss of a breast or a limb. But some losses are invisible to others, such as a loss of energy, the painful uncertainty of tomorrow, or the loss of trust in your body. You may look perfectly normal, yet still see yourself as broken in some way.

> *"Losing bowel and bladder function as well as sexual sensation rocked my whole sense of self — as a woman and in my work in the world. I am still struggling to maintain my dignity in the face of the shame these physical losses bring me. I am much better now than four years ago, when I was filled with despair. It has taken me a long time to learn to live positively despite my disabilities."*
>
> — Mary-Lou, 46 years old, lymphoma, 4-year survivor

How do you begin to re-own your body? Some survivors wear their scars boldly as badges of courage. They are proud to display them and announce to others how they attained them. But others are shy and embarrassed, concealing their scars beneath clothing and bandages, concocting stories of how they resulted from a childhood injury or steering the conversation to another topic. Still others honour their scars with beautiful tattoos, grapevines symbolizing harvest and abundance or flowering tree branches that represent growth and beauty.

> *"I went through a phase after treatment where I wanted to show my scars from surgery and treatment to everyone who was interested. But now I'm okay with my body and I don't need to reveal my battle scars to anyone. They're my scars now, just for me, so that I will remember the experience."*
>
> — Michaela, 26 years old, ovarian cancer, 3-year survivor

How do you reconcile the newly reassembled view of yourself? As a survivor you must re-own your body — both how you see it and how you imagine others perceive it. The process will be different for everyone, and how much time it takes will vary. Some survivors spend their entire lives integrating a new body image into their sense of self. Though the process may be fraught with self-doubt and avoidance, with frustration and discomfort, it remains an inevitable and important part of recovery. You are left with this home for your soul: learning to accept it (even one small part at a time), move into it and get comfortable with it again are important steps in how you will progress.

LEARNING TO TRUST AGAIN

If you have always had a healthy lifestyle, you might feel that your body betrayed you by developing cancer. You exercised regularly, ate healthy foods, and took good care of yourself in the belief that this would guarantee you a healthy life. The arrival of cancer came as a terrible shock. How could this happen to you?

Worse, while the cancer was growing inside you, you had no idea it was there. You wonder how you could have been so out of touch with your body. Perhaps you feel guilty: was there something more you could have done? You've lost trust in your body, too: why didn't it give you any indication something was wrong?

"I rebelled after treatment finished because I thought I had taken such good care of myself before I was diagnosed, but it didn't seem to help me now. I felt really betrayed by my body. I gained weight during chemotherapy and was thrown into menopause where I gained even more weight. I had a mastectomy and ended up with lymphedema in my right arm which swells to the size of a grapefruit. I thought, to hell with this, if it hits people who try to behave, who eat well, exercise, and don't smoke, then forget it. I became a rebel. I ate anything I wanted and I didn't do any exercise. My motto was eat, drink, and be merry. It was a major loss of innocence. I didn't think I should have to face my mortality at such a young age and

with two children under the age of five. I was rebelling because it was my way of getting control of my life. I was also angry at the whole experience. I felt my healthy lifestyle before the cancer had failed me.

"After five years I realized that I was going to make it after all. It turns out my rebellion had been all about dying. If I was going to die, I didn't want to deprive myself of chocolate and bacon and cheese. I started to think maintaining my health is important after all, and I started exercising again, watched my diet, and of course vanity also comes into play. I wanted to look good again."

— Marie-Claire, 35 years old, breast cancer, 6-year survivor

The other side of the coin belongs to those who feel they betrayed their own bodies, whether through smoking, lack of exercise or too much stress. They believe they let their bodies down, not the other way around. Some survivors carry an enormous load of guilt because of this.

"I didn't eat well, I didn't exercise, and I didn't manage my stress at all. I should have seen the doctor sooner; I was careless. I think my body has done a tremendous job living with me."

— Tom, 52 years old, bladder cancer, 2-year survivor

People at different life stages tend to have different views on this subject. As you get older, you begin to accept that your body will not always perform the way it did when you were 20. Illness of all kinds might strike. When it does, many people come to accept it not as a betrayal by the body but as a wounding or weakening of the body that requires time and attention to mend.

Re-owning your body after cancer involves developing a new attitude that goes beyond appearance and image. Rather than failing you, your body has sustained you despite the threat of cancer and the risks of treatment. You might even find that you're grateful your body has held up during all you've gone through. Its healing capabilities are astounding: wounds close, edema lessens, scars shrink. Your body has many things to teach you. Despite your fatigue or despair, it perseveres and carries you through to recovery.

"My body amazed me. I watched it heal, bit by bit. The radiation burn less-ened, my hair grew back, my appetite returned. It seemed like a miracle."
— Terry, 36 years old, leukemia, 6-month survivor

Trust is the cornerstone of any relationship, including your relationship with yourself. Once it has been shaken or betrayed, it is hard to restore. When we feel that we can't trust anymore there's a greyness to life. Our hearts become hard and inflexible and our minds doubt all that we know. Learning to trust again takes time. It will come only when you look inside and begin to believe in your body's instincts and your mind's ability to make choices that are good for you. You start to listen to the signs that your body sends when it needs nourishment or rest. You trust that the inner resources you possess will guide you through the challenges. Slowly you regain confidence in your ability to heal, and you come to expect that you can, once again, trust that you'll be okay whatever comes your way. You can get through the challenges that arise, and you have the inner strength to do so.

"I didn't know when I'd be 'out of the woods,' so I never wanted to recon-nect with my body again. I could see it going through the motions, but I wasn't a part of it. I felt I couldn't afford to get close and then find out the cancer was back. But slowly I found myself turning towards my body, want-ing to mother it like I did my children. Eventually we came to a place of understanding and mutual respect, an intimacy not shared before."
— Consuella, 58 years old, colorectal cancer, 1-year survivor

Like Consuella, some survivors find in the end that cancer has brought them closer to their bodies. They develop a new awareness, an ability to listen to physical messages and make new connections. They are no longer strangers to their bodies; instead they see themselves as keepers of the life force housed within.

 SELF SCAN QUESTIONS 1, 2, 3, 4 AND 5 *(see page 99)*

SIDE EFFECTS: THE UNEXPECTED EXTRA

Twenty-five years ago, little consideration was given to the side effects of cancer treatment. Survivors just considered themselves lucky to be alive. But as more and more people survive cancer, researchers are paying attention to the short- and long-term physical effects of the various types of cancer treatments.

In *A Cancer Survivor's Almanac*, Dr. Fitzhugh Mullen emphasizes cancer's significance in a person's life: "Survivorship is not some club you join after several months of treatment — or after five years or ten years. Rather, survivorship is lifelong, beginning with the diagnosis of cancer and continuing for the balance of one's life." (1)

Cancer is now considered a chronic disease, like heart disease or diabetes. For many, it is a disease that can be managed rather than being cured outright. As more and more people survive, it's about living with cancer and making the necessary adjustments to deal with its side effects.

Even when your treatment is over, your risk for side effects remains. While cancer treatments are meant to kill cancer cells, they can also damage your healthy cells (such as hair and mouth cells). Most of your healthy cells will return to normal after treatment, but this may take time — and unfortunately, the length of time is different for everyone. The standard rule of thumb is that it will take you as long as the total duration of your treatment to feel well again. You will see positive changes with each passing week, but full recovery may be slow.

The side effects you experience may be acute (meaning they are short-lived), long-term (meaning they appear during treatment and persist for some period of time after treatment ends) or late (meaning that they occur months or even years after treatment has been completed).

Some common physical side effects of cancer treatment include:

- Fatigue
- Sleep disturbances
- Pain
- Changes in appetite

- Inability to return to previous physical activities
- Hair loss
- Weight changes — increase in or excessive loss of weight
- Mouth sores, dental or other mouth problems
- For women, changes in menstrual cycle, hot flashes, early menopause
- Bowel changes — constipation or diarrhea
- Numbness or tingling in the hands or feet
- Skin changes
- Joint soreness or arthritic changes
- Sexual problems

Some people do not experience any side effects during or after treatment, while others can have many. Most acute and long-term effects lessen with time. Many late effects can be easily managed, but others pose more serious problems, and some may even be life-threatening. In this book we have room to address only the most common physical side effects for survivors, but we encourage you to find out more about the potential side effects and risk factors for developing late effects associated with your type of cancer and treatment. It is very important that you share any symptoms you're experiencing with your doctor and other members of your health care team, so that they can provide the necessary help and support. If you are not already working with a health care professional, find someone you trust and begin gathering information. Chances are your side effects can be treated.

Fatigue

If you suffer from fatigue, you are not alone. Cancer survivors say that of all the problems they face, fatigue is the most prevalent, and it can often be debilitating. Fatigue afflicts the majority of cancer patients at some point. While many healthy people experience periods of low energy, the fatigue that follows cancer treatments is a real medical condition that, unfortunately, can continue for months or even years after therapy ends.

Cancer-related fatigue (CRF) includes a complex set of symptoms. Unlike regular tiredness, CRF is unpredictable and can impair your day-to-day activities. Survivors have described CRF as "a wall of fatigue," "bone weary tiredness," and "whole body exhaustion." If you do experience CRF, you may notice variations in how the fatigue presents itself. You might feel only a bit low in energy one day but unable to get off the couch the next. You might experience brief periods of intermittent fatigue, or your fatigue might appear daily and last for several months.

"The exhaustion lasted a year before I felt like my old self again. I never knew fatigue like the kind I experienced that first year."
— John, 57 years old, prostate cancer, 3-year survivor

Cancer-related fatigue can show up as acute or chronic fatigue. Acute, or short-term, fatigue is intense, peaks near the end of cancer treatment and gradually reduces with time. It does improve with a good night's sleep, a healthy diet, and regular physical activity. But don't be fooled: recovery from acute fatigue can be slow.

Chronic fatigue is unusual, excessive and constant. It is not relieved by rest, and it persists over time. Besides feeling tired, you may also experience irritability, memory changes, concentration difficulties, depression, weakness, decreased sexual desire, and a general loss of interest in daily activities. Extra effort is required to perform simple everyday activities, and even some of those can become impossible. You may have problems participating in household tasks such as vacuuming and preparing meals. Even climbing stairs or showering becomes a chore.

Whatever shape your fatigue takes, it can interfere with, even impair, your ability to function in daily life. How long will it last? There's no definitive answer. For most people, CRF gets better over time. But for some, the decrease in energy may last for years. Many survivors feel frustrated when fatigue lasts longer than they think it should. It may help to know that, as a rule, the more intense and prolonged your treatment, the longer its after-effects. One oncology nurse counsels, "Don't expect to have your full energy back for at least one year after your treatment is complete. If you expect it to return in two or three months, you will be disappointed." (2)

Although fatigue is common, it is not a topic often discussed between survivors and their doctors. Survivors may not mention their fatigue, assuming it is a normal part of recovery and nothing can be done about it, or not wanting to bother their doctor with this "small" problem. After all, they're still alive. But in most cases, fatigue can be managed by changing your lifestyle and medications in combination with learning energy-conservation techniques. Always keep in mind that the factors that contribute to your fatigue may be completely different from those of another survivor. Eventually, most survivors come to respect their fatigue. They become aware of the consequences of pushing through it. They learn to work with the ebb and flow of energy and rest.

 SELF SCAN QUESTIONS 6, 7, 8, 9, 10 AND 11 *(see page 99)*

Sleep Disturbances

A restful night's sleep is essential to our well-being and our ability to function in daily life. But many survivors experience a change in their sleep patterns due to the worry and fear that accompany a diagnosis of cancer. Financial worries, work concerns, and self doubts also keep us awake. Upsetting dreams or nightmares about the cancer experience may cause sleepless nights. Physical considerations can also intrude: you may have to take medications at varying times, or aches and pains might awaken you from a sound sleep. Side effects such as changes in bowel and bladder habits or incontinence affect your ability to get a good night's sleep, as does a change in activity levels during the day.

Insomnia can leave you feeling short-tempered, irritable, impatient or on edge. It can also impair memory, reaction times and productivity at work. Lack of sleep affects not only your energy level but also your mental functioning day to day. When you don't get enough sleep, you can't handle stress very well, either, which impairs the body's ability to heal.

Good-quality sleep is an essential component of recovery. Maybe you need to give yourself permission to rest or nap during the day (for no more than 20 minutes) when you're feeling sluggish. Alternatively, you may need to stop napping three to four times a day and aim instead for one good night's sleep. Everybody has different sleep needs; what works for one person may not work for another. Learn what you need to feel good during the day, stick to a regular schedule and address the issues that keep you awake at night. It is also possible to get medication to break the sleepless cycle and let you return to a regular pattern. See your doctor if sleeplessness persists.

 SELF SCAN QUESTIONS 12 AND 13 *(see page 100)*

Pain

Pain is both the warning system and the protective mechanism that enables an individual to defend the integrity of his or her body. One in three cancer survivors experiences pain. It comes in many forms and differing intensities. Every experience of pain is unique, since we all have different pain thresholds. Pain can be dull, aching, sharp, constant, intermittent, mild, moderate, or severe. It can vary from hour to hour. Pain can be a minor annoyance, or it can be incapacitating.

When you are uncertain about your health you tend to feel anxious. Unfortunately, anxiety and pain build upon each other. As one increases, the other follows suit, until you have a spiral of physical and emotional turmoil that leaves you unable to function.

> *"Dealing with my back pain occupied my whole day. I had to adjust my work schedule and the time I spent with friends to accommodate the amount of pain I was feeling. I wasn't able to tolerate the many hours needed to work full-time, and I missed many social events because I couldn't count on feeling well enough to stay for the entire outing."*
> — Tammy, 32 years old, lung cancer, 3-year survivor

Many survivors are reluctant to admit they experience pain. They may feel pain is to be expected, or they don't want to be seen as complainers by their doctors. They may worry that pain is a sign of recurrence. They may fear becoming addicted to pain medications. But as harsh as pain can be at times, it can also be relieved in the majority of patients.

It's important to monitor your pain over a period of time — several times a day for several weeks — so that you can provide your health care team with the information they need to develop an appropriate treatment plan. This record is referred to as a pain diary. The questions on pain in this chapter's Self Scan will help you get started on your pain diary if you need to create one.

 SELF SCAN QUESTIONS 14, 15, 16 AND 17 *(see page 100)*

Nutrition: What to Eat?

The food we eat nourishes us and is the building block for a healthy mind and body. Many of us have an ongoing struggle with food. We know what is good for us, but we don't always eat that way. After experiencing cancer, almost everyone wants to know what they should and should not eat — what promotes healing and what impedes it.

Weight gain and weight loss issues may become apparent as well once treatment has ended. A weight gain of five to fifteen pounds after chemotherapy can be due to the side effects of certain drugs or to eating habits developed to deal with nausea (frequent snacking or many small meals throughout the day). A change in metabolism may affect how easy it is to lose those extra pounds. Excessive weight loss creates its own problems, and it needs to be addressed immediately so that other health concerns do not arise.

Many survivors report that their relationship with food changed after the cancer experience. Some rebelled and ate anything they wanted; others bargained with their food and their nutritionists ("I'll eat three vegetables a day if I can still have my two glasses of red wine at night"). Still others jumped into strict new diets in an attempt to control the disease. Many survivors become more conscious of the relationship between seeing their food as nourishment and what it takes to heal and stay healthy.

As a survivor, you'll find that everyone has an opinion about what you should and shouldn't eat. Perhaps the hardest issue is sorting through the endless supply of information on dietary and nutritional approaches to cancer therapy. Conflicting information comes out almost weekly on what's good to eat and what's considered harmful. The answers vary from one expert to the next. It's confusing and upsetting, since you know that your diet will influence the healing process.

 SELF SCAN QUESTIONS 18, 19 AND 20 *(see page 100)*

Physical and Leisure Activity: What's Changed?

After cancer, you may be unsure of the best way to get moving again. How much exertion is healthy? Will you hurt yourself? Many survivors have been told to rest. You may worry about your fluctuating energy levels. You fear your stamina is not what it once was; your immune system has been weakened, and your heart, muscles and bones may be vulnerable.

It is true that after cancer treatment you may not be able to return right away to your previous activities. Even your daily routine of housework and self-care may prove challenging. But new medical evidence shows that a return to physical activity is essential for overcoming the negative effects of cancer treatment.

Before beginning any physical activity after cancer, it is important to speak to your physician or a trained exercise specialist. There are newly emerging guidelines on aerobic exercise, weight training, and other physical activities that can rebuild (for some, build for the first time) cardiovascular fitness and muscle strength and endurance. Learning the safest way to begin rebuilding your body while minimizing potential side effects helps you get back the activities you love.

You also need to stay in touch with your own needs. Those who are fast movers may need to give themselves permission to slow down and enjoy a more peaceful type of exercise, such as yoga, that includes breathing and body awareness. Others need the motivation to get off the couch, so their job is to start walking every day.

Once you decide to return to the activities you love, you may need to rework your previous tried-and-true systems.

"My husband and I love to camp, but the first time I went camping with my new colostomy bag was a whole new experience for me. It took some

time to work out the kinks, but in the end all was good. We go several
times a year now."

— Patsy, 47 years old, colon cancer, 5-year survivor

Some survivors, such as those who have had lymph nodes removed from under an arm or in the groin area, may have limitations that prevent a full return to a sport or activity right away. Breast cancer survivors may choose to wear a compression sleeve to help prevent lymphedema, or swelling, from developing in the arm. A slow but sure return to your daily activities around the house will help you regain a sense of normalcy. Returning to the sports and leisure activities you love, armed with knowledge and guided by your health care provider, will make you feel better and help you to regain energy, strength and stamina.

 SELF SCAN QUESTIONS 21 AND 22 *(see page 100 and 101)*

Sexual Problems

After cancer, you may experience changes in your sex life. A large percentage of women who have had long-term treatment for breast or reproductive organ cancer and many men treated for prostate or testicular cancer report experiencing sexual problems. Changes in sexuality can be yet another blow to recovering your sense of self, and these can add more stress to the relationship you have with your partner.

Sexual issues experienced by women following surgery, chemotherapy or radiation treatment include pain during intercourse, loss of libido, difficulty achieving orgasm, menopausal symptoms, infertility, loss of self esteem and poor body image. For men, problems with impotence, incontinence, and premature ejaculation can affect confidence and self-esteem.

"We had a good sex life before the cancer, but now my problems of incon-
tinence and irregular erections have put a real damper on it. We're never
sure what will happen next. We pretend it doesn't matter, but it does."

— Sam, 58 years old, prostate cancer, 3-year survivor

Your body image may be affected by hair loss, scars, loss of your sexual body parts, disfigurement, changes in weight, unusual and uncomfortable sensations in your body, and mood swings. You may believe you are now unattractive, or you may be convinced your partner no longer finds you desirable. Perhaps you don't like the look of your new body or you fear the way your partner may perceive it. All of this will have a negative impact on sex, making it uncomfortable and embarrassing.

People with ostomies after colon or rectal surgery may feel ashamed of the changes to their bodies, fearful that their partners will reject them, or worried that an accident will occur.

> *"The colostomy makes noise and smells and it's embarrassing — I just want to reject it. It feels like an attachment, not a part of my body. Sex makes me very emotional; I often cry."*
> — Nhien, 52 years old, colorectal cancer, 2-year survivor

Both you and your partner may be uncertain about how to proceed. You almost lost each other; now you're both holding on tightly. Pleasurable physical contact and the excitement you once shared can seem like a distant dream, but if you avoid each other you will exacerbate the doubt you are both feeling. Good communication is essential to overcoming these new fears. Just remember that sorting through such difficult emotions takes time.

You may also experience a change in your femininity or masculinity. Walking into a lingerie store for the first time after having had breast cancer can be overwhelming. Many women are reduced to tears when they try on a new bra, imagining other women in the store with perky, beautiful breasts while they're left with one breast and scars.

> *"My husband and I have only made love a few times since my mastectomy. I feel uneasy about the scars and worry he's not comfortable with them either. I don't feel as sexy as I used to; it's going to take time to get there again. If I don't feel at ease with my new body, how will he?"*
> — Crystal, 49 years old, breast cancer, 4-month survivor

Men report feeling less masculine because they've lost a testicle or their prostate gland and are having trouble getting or maintaining an erection.

Loss of libido is one of the most frequently reported problems affecting sexual intimacy. It's normal to have a decrease in or a loss of sexual desire due to all the other changes you are going through. Fatigue and pain can decrease sexual desire, and when fear is all-consuming sexuality gets put on the back burner. It's hard to be in the mood when you are preoccupied with just making it through the day.

Sometimes sexual problems also have emotional causes such as depression, grief at losing the intimacy you once shared with your partner, and fear of rejection. Anger, blame, guilt and self-doubt may also get expressed in the bedroom, resulting in one partner withdrawing from the other.

Reclaiming your sexuality is an important part of recovering your sense of self. If you have sexual concerns or problems, address them with your health care provider. Trained sexuality counsellors can be invaluable at this time, and seeking out a counsellor who shares your cultural background might be worthwhile. In some cases, sexual dysfunction slowly returns to normal on its own after surgery or radiation; in other cases, drugs or other therapies can be used to successfully treat it. What can seem awkward at first may forge a deeper connection with your partner over time.

 SELF SCAN QUESTIONS 23 AND 24 *(see page 101)*

TIME HEALS

Reconnecting with your body can be a slow and difficult process, but it is important to remember that time is a healing balm. Your body is capable of healing itself. Side effects will lessen. Eventually, you will move towards a place of accepting your new physical self. Move forward with patience and compassion into this new territory of recovery, and soon it will feel like home.

SELF SCAN NUMBER 1: ASSESSING YOUR BODY

Your relationship with your body

1. How would you describe your relationship with your body prior to cancer?

2. Since your treatment ended, how are you responding to your body — have you turned away from it or embraced it more fully?

3. How do you treat your scars from cancer (internal and external): like a badge of courage? as something to acknowledge privately? as something to keep hidden from view, from both yourself and others?

4. Do you feel that your body has betrayed you? Or do you feel that you have betrayed it? How so?

5. What changes have you observed as your body is healing? What do you need to do in order to see your body as a healer?

Assessing your fatigue

6. Rate your current level of fatigue on a scale of 0-10 (with 0 being no fatigue and 10 being the worst fatigue you've ever experienced).

7. When did you begin to experience fatigue, and how has it progressed since your diagnosis?

8. How long does the fatigue last?

9. What makes it worse? What eases it?

10. Describe how fatigue affects your daily life. Are you able to do the activities you did prior to the cancer? If not, describe the ways in which fatigue interferes with:

    • activities you enjoy
    • work duties and responsibilities
    • your ability to visit or socialize
    • family roles and responsibilities.

11. What do you do when the fatigue occurs? Do you fight it? Face it? Are there repercussions later? Do you have a plan for how to work with the fatigue when it happens?

Assessing your sleep habits

12. How have your sleep patterns changed since treatment ended? Do you get enough sleep to be alert and productive, or are you sluggish throughout the day?

13. If you're having trouble sleeping, begin monitoring your sleep patterns. What wakes you up: bad dreams? needing to go to the bathroom? fear? pain?

Assessing your pain

14. Rate your current level of pain on a scale of 0-10 (with 0 being no pain and 10 being the worst pain you've ever experienced).

15. Describe both what the pain feels like (sharp, dull and achy, burning, throbbing, steady, etc.) and the exact places where you experience it. Note whether the pain stays in one place or moves around.

16. When do you feel the pain? Note when it starts, how long it lasts, and whether it gets better or worse at certain times of the day or night. Is there anything you do that makes it better or worse?

17. Be specific in describing how the pain affects your daily life. Does it stop you from working? doing household chores? seeing your friends and family? going out and having fun? pain does not have to be excruciating to have a negative impact on your life.

Your relationship with food

18. What role did food play in your life before your cancer diagnosis?

19. Do you think that food can be a source of healing? If yes, how so?

20. What food choices have you made (eliminated or added) because of cancer?

Your activity level

21. Are there daily activities you were able to do prior to the cancer that you can no longer do? If so, list them. Which activities can you still do but less frequently or for a shorter duration? (Vacuuming, lifting dishes overhead, doing household chores, climbing stairs, and taking care of yourself are all possible examples).

22. Are there any leisure or recreational activities you were able to do prior to the cancer that you can no longer do? If so, list them. Which activities can you still do but less frequently or for a shorter duration? (For example, walking around the block instead of hiking for the day, golfing nine instead of eighteen holes, playing fewer games of tennis.)

Your sexuality

23. How has cancer affected your sex life? In what ways have you tried to accommodate the changes that have occurred? Are you satisfied with how you are managing these changes, or do you feel you need help?

24. Has your sense of femininity or masculinity changed since the cancer? How?

CHAPTER SIX

What's on Your Mind: Assessing Your Thoughts and Emotions

"Emotional pain — when you are hurting on the inside — was even harder to heal than the physical pain. I swallowed all my hurts and held my breath, because after all everyone has done for me, if I complain, I feel like the bad guy."

— Saul, 43 years old, lymphoma, 3-month survivor

"I'm learning to recognize my emotional ups and downs and to be gentle with them. It's a combination of acknowledging, staying connected to and then building on what I'm honestly feeling. It is a balancing act; happy, sad, angry and confused, they all have to be there."

— Nancy, 51 years old, breast cancer, 1-year survivor

Cancer may be a disease of the body, but most survivors find it leaves emotional scars that are even more difficult to heal than the physical ones. Often the emotional turmoil doesn't begin until your treatment has ended and you have time to sort out what has happened to you. That's when you suddenly find yourself on an emotional roller-coaster that takes you to the heights of joy and gratitude, only to plunge you down the next moment into fear, depression and guilt.

"When I was diagnosed with cancer, I pretended nothing had happened.
I never missed a day at work while I was in treatment. I thought I was
strong and in control of my life. But after treatment ended, I went into a
deep funk for six months."

— Bjorn, 53 years old, melanoma, 8-month survivor

Life brings many pressures of its own — financial demands, familial responsibilities, expectations at work. Survivors must bear the added burden of recovering from treatment side effects and living with the fear of a recurrence. Many try at first to deny or hide their feelings of anger, sadness, or fear. You can feel overwhelmed and helpless when such strong emotions wash over you. You may hope these unresolved feelings will work themselves out, but the contrary seems to be true: ignored feelings call even louder, until you can't help but listen to them.

The Self Scan at the end of this chapter will help you become more aware of the range of emotions you might be experiencing, and of the attitudes and beliefs that inform those feelings.

ATTITUDES AND BELIEFS

Your *attitude* is how you think about and relate to a situation. We form our attitudes from our experiences. Reinforced by internal dialogue — self talk — our attitudes can distort facts and alter truth by attributing a particular meaning to an event and sending us messages about both the event and ourselves.

Attitudes are powerful forces. They influence not only our orientation in life, but also our health — both physical and mental. If we perceive a circumstance or situation to be positive, we welcome it, or at least do not detach or push it away. Conversely, if something is disturbing or disruptive to us, we can experience any number of negative emotions and uncomfortable physical sensations.

For large portions of our daily lives, we function on automatic, barely conscious of our own thoughts, opinions and ideas. Cancer tends to flip that autopilot switch off. Cancer survivors speak of experiencing an attitude adjustment as they begin to rethink how they want to live their lives. Healing from within involves adopting attitudes and patterns of thought that help you to renew or restore your health.

> *"From cancer I learned a lot about the power of attitude. You don't have to be a victim; you can change the way you think. I began to think of myself as a warrior. I wanted to be strong and healthy, not sick and dependent."*
> — Brandon, 60 years old, prostate cancer, 1-year survivor

Beliefs are the ideas that we hold to be true about life. Most of our actions and interactions are governed by our belief systems, often without our knowing it. Our beliefs and assumptions shape our actions, and they affect our ability to listen to and interact with others. Beliefs imbue our lives with meaning and serve as an internal compass, guiding us through confusing or difficult situations. However, some of our beliefs can become obstacles to living well.

In his book *After the Ecstasy, the Laundry*, Jack Kornfield writes, "Central to the stories we tell are the fixed beliefs we have about ourselves ... These patterns of thought, together with the contractions of the body and heart, create a limited sense of self ... our life is simply one of habit and reaction." (1)

Often, our beliefs are passed on to us from our families. They become incorporated into our lives without much thought and remain largely untested. Many of us were taught at an early age, for example, to put aside our own instincts and trust in external voices of authority (parents, teachers, clergy, doctors, and so on).

The beliefs we inherit from our families influence how we see the world and what kind of choices we make. There are daily examples of how suspicions, prejudices, even hatred can be passed down from generation to generation. Beliefs that repeatedly trigger feelings of guilt, shame, anger, anxiety and fear can run through families as if genetically coded. However, once we realize that we have adopted a belief that hinders us in some way, we can take control of our lives by choosing to believe something different.

Examining inherited beliefs about illness can be very important for survivors.

In some families, only the doctor could pronounce you sick. No matter how bad you felt, unless you were so sick a doctor had to be called — off to school you went. In other families, being sick meant receiving extra love and attention from your parents. You felt supported and taken care of, trusting that everything would work out. Your early experiences have taught you either to suffer in silence or to honour your body's need for rest and time to heal.

> *"In my family, if anything happened, you got back in the game as soon as possible. You certainly didn't take time off and sit around feeling sorry for yourself. That ingrained belief made it very difficult for me to take the time I needed to recover."*
>
> — Norma, 54 years old, oral cancer, 3-year survivor

Our beliefs can stem from even limited experiences. If your neighbour died of cancer and so did your grandfather, you may unconsciously believe that all people with cancer die. Even though you've survived, you expect the worst and cannot trust that living well with cancer is truly possible.

> *"My mom died of cancer in her fifties, and it was a very traumatic death for me. I was in my early twenties, and our family didn't deal with it at all. She didn't talk about dying, and we didn't talk to each other about her dying. In our family, if anything bad happened, we just pretended it didn't happen. I learned to keep my feelings buried."*
>
> — Giselle, 51 years old, colorectal cancer, 9-month survivor

On the other hand, if you've known family members or friends who were diagnosed with cancer and recovered well, you may believe it's a disease from which you will emerge victorious.

As a cancer survivor, you may come into recovery with pre-existing attitudes and beliefs that support and enhance your recovery. Or you may see cancer as an opportunity for increasing your self-awareness, self-knowledge, and empowerment. Cancer can become the turning point in changing your mind, breaking free from attitudes and beliefs that no longer serve you well.

BELIEFS ARE CHANGEABLE

When your treatment ends, you will rarely be told you're cured; instead, your doctor may tell you that you are in remission. Your beliefs about your current state of health will influence the way you approach your recovery. If you've seen others go through a painful and lengthy recovery, that may affect what you believe is possible for yourself. Such negativity can sabotage your healing. What happened to someone else is not necessarily what will happen to you. Even if you have the same type and stage of cancer, your unique background and experiences will determine your recovery process.

Through our work with cancer survivors, we have observed five major beliefs that positively influence healing:

- Belief in yourself
- Belief in your treatment
- Belief in your health care team
- Belief in your body's ability to heal
- Belief in your own ability to move forward and deal with both loss and change

Positive role models can also serve as an inspiration. Maybe you've seen family members, friends or work colleagues go through cancer and come out stronger and more alive. Survivor groups can provide highly positive role models, too. Through such activities as fly fishing, mountain trekking, participating on a dragon boat team, or volunteering at the local cancer centre, survivors can demonstrate to one another — and the world — that there is life after cancer.

 SELF SCAN QUESTIONS 1, 2 AND 3 *(see page 128)*

MEMORY AND CONCENTRATION

Survivors often complain of "being lost in a fog." "I just forgot the word," some say or "I don't seem to be able to concentrate like before."

The term "chemobrain" or "chemofog" is used by cancer survivors to describe the changes in memory and in the ability to focus or concentrate that may result from chemotherapy treatments. In medical language, these effects are referred to as "cognitive deficits" or "declining neuropsychological functioning." It can be frustrating and alarming during recovery to find yourself forgetful or unable to multi-task as you could before the cancer.

> *"I joked with my oncologist during my one-year follow-up visit that if he had advised me that I would experience memory loss and cloudy thinking as a side-effect of my chemo, I don't remember!"*
> — Samantha, 46 years old, breast cancer, 1-year survivor

A major challenge for survivors with ongoing memory and concentration difficulties is sorting out whether these difficulties are due to the chemotherapy or to other factors. Fatigue, disturbed sleep, menopause, aging, medication, stress and depression can also cause cognitive dysfunction. Whatever their absolute cause, these cognitive changes are real, and they can be distressing. It is reassuring to know that chemobrain is not usually a permanent condition, and these deficits usually improve with time. See your physician with any concerns you may have.

 SELF SCAN QUESTION 4 *(see page 128)*

THE EMOTIONAL ROLLERCOASTER

Feelings arise from the voices in our heads and hearts. They give our lives colour, whether it is the yellow sunshine of joy or the blackness of depression. While they can be problematic, feelings are not problems in themselves. Often there is a good reason that we feel as we do. Unfortunately, many of us have been taught to suppress or dismiss our feelings, because they are illogical or uncomfortable for others to deal with.

"You can't move through a feeling that you're not allowed to have. If you have negative thoughts of fear, grief, or dread, you must be allowed to have them, to get through them. People tell me to be happy, be positive, not to let myself get down. But such advice doesn't help you move forward at all."

— Mikhail, 71 years old, prostate cancer, 3-year survivor

After cancer, you may feel as if the emotional ground beneath your feet is shifting. The post-treatment range of emotions is vast and vacillating: one moment you may feel cheated, the next, grateful to be alive. One day may bring feelings of confidence; with the next comes despair. While times of transition are often characterized by conflicting feelings, the intensity or rawness of your post-treatment emotions may come as a surprise.

Emotions that are unchallenged or unwanted can, at best, wrap us in a fog and, at worst, create severe anxiety and depression. All emotions need to be acknowledged. When you're completing this chapter's Self Scan, it's important to step back from your feelings in order to look at them objectively, curiously, and without judgement.

Some of the common emotional side effects of cancer treatment include:

- Anger and resentment
- Depression
- Embarrassment and shame
- Fear
- Gratitude and love
- Guilt and blame
- Joy and happiness
- Sadness and grief

Our feelings declare themselves in a variety of ways, and each of us responds to them uniquely. However, there is some common ground. Anxiety, fear, and uncertainty about your current and future capabilities can trigger guilt, resentment and a loss of confidence. Another factor that can affect your emotional recovery is whether or not you have attached any shame, guilt or blame to your cancer experience. Such strong negative emotions can wreak havoc on your sense of self.

"I should never have laid in the sun, or smoked or drank during my teen years. Now I'm beating myself up because of my past and wondering if I'll ever be healthy again."

— Roberto, 24 years old, lung cancer, 1-year survivor

During treatment, many survivors feel they must be strong, so they keep their fears and emotions tucked in. In the unstructured quiet times, after the treatments end, those feelings are unleashed. Now that the fight is over, all the repressed frustration, resentment, relief and gratitude can come to the surface in an overwhelming rush.

"During my illness, I was the strong one for my friends and family, always the one with the positive attitude. But after treatment, I lost it. I really fell apart. I fluctuated between being angry and terrified that I would die, and happy and grateful for being alive. These big emotional changes drained me and left me wondering what was happening to me."

— Lynn, 48 years old, leukemia, 2-year survivor

The responses of well-meaning family and friends may encourage you to stifle negative emotions. People say, "You must be so relieved the cancer is behind you" or "You've been so brave," and you think, *I'd better keep up a good front; I'd better not let them down.* You begin to suppress your fears, trying to forget about the experience in an effort to move on. But don't let the opinions of others stop you from getting the help you need to recover. Friends and family may be afraid to face thoughts of your mortality as well as their own, resulting in discomfort or an inability to listen to your fears.

Your emotions will not stay pushed aside, and acknowledging and expressing them will help you in your recovery. Emotions rise to the surface and then recede, like a constant tide: you are meant to feel them, not keep them at bay. They will continue to change by themselves.

"I used to repress the sadness and loneliness that welled up in my throat because I believed it was a sign of strength not to cry. I kept hoping that in time it would take care of itself. My friends would tell me, 'Don't cry, it'll be alright.' But my feelings grew stronger until I couldn't ignore them anymore."

— Juliet, 54 years old, ovarian cancer, 2-year survivor

Each of us must work through our feelings in our own way and in our own time. Awakening to your emotions doesn't mean you must judge them. Instead, it means you observe them and gently allow them to move through you. Needless to say, we are better able to do this on some days than on others.

As you move through the questions in the Self Scan, try to be open to the feelings that present themselves. Recognize that you may feel emotionally vulnerable right now. This is an opportunity to practise being compassionate towards yourself.

"I am 'relearning' about myself, and it requires so much patience. I'm certainly more compassionate towards others, and in many ways I have also become more compassionate towards myself."

— Pashada, 49 years old, head/neck cancer, 1-year survivor

 SELF SCAN QUESTIONS 5 AND 6 *(see page 128)*

DIFFICULT EMOTIONS

Most survivors find themselves grappling with difficult emotions as they recover. While there are as many different emotions as there are people, the following feelings are the ones cancer survivors mention most often.

Anger

Anger is our most primitive emotion, and sometimes our most obvious one. Anger arises when something or someone, either physically or psychologically, gets in the way of something we intensely desire. Anger can also be a response to sudden and unexpected change. Anger comes from feeling hurt or wounded or fearful, but it can manifest in a variety of ways, including intolerance, rebellion, resentment, bitterness, hostility, envy, or withdrawal and depression.

Anger is a strong emotion, and one that takes many survivors by surprise. Some people are angry at the cancer: it has taken so many lives and has stolen both time and happiness from them. Present and future plans have been destroyed, and people have been left feeling infuriated.

"While my buddy was hiking around having a great time, I was home reading about free radicals and how to prevent a recurrence."
— Benjamin, 28 years old, melanoma, 5-month survivor

Some survivors are angry about something that happened — or didn't happen — during diagnosis or treatment. They weren't treated well by medical staff; the x-rays missed the cancer the first time around; they were told about the cancer in an abrupt and uncaring manner. Others remain angry at the unfairness of their diagnosis. They had taken good care of themselves, done the right things, and lived healthily, so why did they get the disease? Still others are shocked to find that their family's life and routines have carried on without them. Other people's lives have to continue, of course, but sometimes survivors feel they have been scarcely missed. Many survivors feel irritable or fall into bad moods they can't always explain.

"I needed to be angry about what had happened and the time I'd lost. It's bitterly disappointing to be living your life and then suddenly, one day, all of these things are taken away. And on top of that, you see that life around you doesn't fall apart without you! Buses keep running, stores are still open, the world keeps on ticking, but my life had come to a grinding halt."
— Rosa, 41 years old, lung cancer, 2-year survivor

Your perspective and priorities may have changed after cancer, too. It's hard to be patient with insignificant things when you have faced death. You feel gratitude and appreciation for life and can be annoyed by the importance others assign to life's little miseries.

"I would get really angry at other people's trite problems. I felt righteous in my anger. I wanted to shout, 'You don't know what I've been through and how hard it was.' Eventually I realized no one can really understand what I went through."

— Ned, 23 years old, osteosarcoma, 1-year survivor

Anger contains energy that needs to go somewhere. Suppressed or bottled-up anger can be a contributing factor in such health issues as hypertension, ulcers and injuries. Whether you are angry at God, disappointed by family or friends, or overcome with envy at what you perceive to be another's easy life, it is important to acknowledge unresolved anger and recognize how it can impede recovery.

"Finally I gave myself permission to be angry. I was angry at my body, angry at the cancer, angry at life. I lost my temper over little things. My family was patient and allowed me to be angry. Eventually I didn't need to be angry anymore."

— Vince, 53 years old, throat cancer, 1-year survivor

Because the negative consequences of anger are noisy and upsetting, it is easy to forget that there is also a positive side to anger. For survivors, anger can be the harbinger that tells you your old self has changed and something new is taking its place. Anger can energize you. It can be the internal motivating force that sparks you to action, including getting the help or care you need to recover. There is a very close relationship between anger and fear; many psychologists believe that most anger has fear at its root. Consequently, anger can be an excellent antidote to fear. As an old adage has it, "Don't get scared, get mad." When we are angered by injustice, or speak up in defence of our values, we feel strong and confident. Righteous anger can also bring with it a greater sense of control. Some survivors use their anger as a kick-start to living a healthier life.

"I turned my anger from a negative to a positive. I wasn't going to let the cancer get the best of me. I started reading about nutrition and exercise

and vitamin supplements and devised a program that would work for me and my lifestyle. Now I feel like a million bucks."

— Herbert, 43 years old, lymphoma, 2-year survivor

The source of your anger may also lie in the past. Unfinished business, old grudges, grievances, and emotional traumas can drain your energy and eat away at your sense of well-being. It is important to face and put to rest issues from the past that are still present and getting in your way. It isn't easy, but addressing these issues is essential to finding peace of mind, whether that involves forgiveness, acceptance or letting go.

"Emotional baggage was my biggie. I had unfinished issues that niggled at me, sapping my energy and putting a cloud over my life. Now I'm getting in touch with all the baggage that I'd been dragging along for so many years. I'm getting help to work through it and am experiencing the joyous release that comes from letting it go."

— Marsha, 45 years old, cervical cancer, 3-year survivor

 SELF SCAN QUESTIONS 7, 8 AND 9 *(see page 128)*

Sadness and Depression

Cancer casts a shadow over life. We tend to label the occurrences in our life as good or bad, and we secretly hope to eliminate the dark times, leaving only the positive times to shine through. However, any accomplished painter must be able to work with both shadow and light. We need our sadness. It is through sadness that we grieve our losses.

To be sad is to "feel blue," to be low in spirit, sorrowful or mournful due to the presence of some form of mental and/or emotional suffering. Feeling sad is the polar opposite of feeling happy. Sadness lessens our vitality and is the cause of our tears. Remorse, regret, loneliness and disappointment are all types of sadness. Grief is deep, profound sadness.

When we experience a loss or a trauma, it's normal and appropriate to feel sad. We miss what we have lost, whether it is a relationship, a bodily function, or our dreams for the future. We have down days when we feel prone to crying, and crying can be a great release. During transition periods, sadness comes and goes. For cancer survivors, sadness is often most intense immediately after treatment ends, when the rushing to various appointments stops and the quiet begins.

There is sorrow at having to face your own mortality, and a deep sadness can underlie life as you realize yours was almost taken away. The changes in your daily routine may make you sad. You may have unhappy memories and feelings of despair as you wrestle with losses, both old and new.

> *"I felt a lot of sadness that first year. In the early days after treatment ended and I realized what was still ahead of me, I cried every day. But with time I found I could put the sadness to one side and carry on with the rest of my life."*
>
> — Marion, 37 years old, breast cancer, 2-year survivor

Depression, however, goes beyond sadness. It is like a black tunnel with no light at the end. Feelings of grief, defeat, hopelessness and anxiety can combine with acute stress reactions such as loss of energy, concentration impairment, pain, sleep disturbance, decreased libido, and changes in appetite to create depression. This insidious disorder can cause you to have an absence of emotion and to withdraw from the world around you. You may feel the joy has gone out of your life. Everything seems negative, and there is little hope for the future.

Studies indicate that a significant percentage of cancer patients meet the criteria for a depressive or anxiety disorder at some point during and/or after treatment. Often the signs and symptoms of depression go undiagnosed and so are not treated.

> *"At about six months after surgery it hit me. I felt sad and powerless to change what was going on. I wasn't healing; I was exhausted and not leaving the house too often. I went into a deep, dark hole and became very depressed."*
>
> — Hazel, 52 years old, ovarian cancer, 2-year survivor

The cancer itself can produce abnormal hormonal reactions, and powerful chemotherapy drugs sometimes cause depressive symptoms. But depression can come from an emotional source such as unresolved anger or guilt or the inability to cope with overwhelming fears. The loss of faith or of hope for the future, as well as feelings of isolation and alienation, all contribute to depression. Survivors have described it as "a dark feeling of helplessness" or "an unshakeable sense of impending doom." There is no zest in life; it all feels grey and flat.

Even if you have a positive attitude and great coping skills, the physical and emotional changes caused by the cancer and its treatments can still cause depression. You can't wish it away, and it doesn't go away on its own. Depression indicates that something is wrong and needs attention. It can have a serious effect on your overall recovery and quality of life if left untreated. Don't suffer in silence. Depression requires medical help and usually responds well to treatment.

> *"Activities I used to enjoy, I no longer wanted to do. I'd make plans and then cancel them. I was weepy and slept a lot. I felt like everything was a struggle. I forced myself to do things when I really wanted to hide and protect myself—from what? From death of course. I remember saying to my husband that I was so sad and he said, 'It's more like you're depressed.' That came as such a shock because I had never been depressed in my life. It was at that point that I realized I needed help."*
>
> — Vera, 56 years old, oral cancer, 3-year survivor

Occasionally, cancer survivors may have a particularly difficult time psychologically. When an individual is exposed to a life-threatening event, injury or illness, it is possible to develop symptoms consistent with a syndrome called post-traumatic stress disorder (PTSD). Although this syndrome is often seen in survivors of war or natural disasters, some cancer survivors may exhibit feelings and behaviours that fit. Experiencing another trauma before your cancer may also make you more vulnerable to PTSD. If you are having persistent recollections or flashbacks, recurrent distressing dreams, intrusive or upsetting thoughts, mood swings, difficulty sleeping and communicating, or intense emotional distress when exposed to cues that resemble an aspect of your trauma, it's important to discuss these with your health care professional.

 SELF SCAN QUESTIONS 10 AND 11 *(see page 128)*

Fear

Fear alerts us to danger. It is a warning system that mobilizes us to protect ourselves. We all live with a variety of fears. There are the subtle, underlying fears such as the fear of looking foolish or of making the wrong decision. Then there are the more intense, overt fears of being alone, losing your job, getting sick, and dying. These fears can bring us to our knees.

Fear wears many disguises: it can manifest itself as unease, worry, anxiety, shyness, indecision, nervousness, dread, aggression, aggrandizing behaviour or feelings of inferiority. It can be strong enough to paralyze us. While fear has a helpful side, it becomes harmful when it is ignored or denied or when it overwhelms us. Fear varies in intensity, type and breadth. While some fears are based on reality, we create other fears ourselves when we focus on the worst that can happen. When fear enters your heart and mind, it is hard to trust the river of ongoing change. Whether you are afraid of the cancer, of dying, or of not living fully in the time you have left, if you cling to fear it can become your constant companion.

> *"The fear has come to land in a deep place. I'm terrified of dying, of leaving my family, of not accomplishing what I want to do. It seems to be always there, hanging over me, threatening me."*
> — Marcus, 43 years old, leukemia, 9-month survivor

Fear is a normal reaction to the diagnosis of cancer. But to be continuously afraid is truly to suffer. Some survivors develop an anxiety disorder that pervades their lives. Times of intense fear are sometimes described as dark nights of the soul, in which we descend into a disorienting, frightening place within ourselves that holds deep and threatening emotions. Many survivors describe the anguish fear has created in their lives and express the need to learn ways to handle it. Family and friends try to be helpful when they tell you not to worry. Unfortunately, the result is that you may suppress your fears, which minimizes your experience. Denying fear rarely makes it go away. And often what's on the surface is only masking the true cause of your fear.

When you acknowledge your fear, you take the first step toward taming it. Entering the state of fear with courage and curiosity can provide an opportunity for you to learn more about yourself. As you move through transition, your fears and how you feel about them will fluctuate from day to day, perhaps hour to hour. To develop coping skills, as well as longer-term adaptive strategies, you must take stock of your fears and try to understand how they affect your life.

Fears common to survivors include:

- Fear of recurrence: Will the cancer come back?
- Fear of stress: If I get stressed out, will the cancer recur? Does stress cause cancer?
- Fear of the unknown: Will the side effects diminish? When will I feel like my old self again? What if I have to face another diagnosis of cancer?
- Fear of the future: How do I live for today and still plan for tomorrow? Will I have a future?
- Fear of change: How will I deal with the changes caused by cancer?
- Fear of dying: Will I die? Will it be painful?
- Fear of not living fully: Will I go back to not living each day to the utmost, not being fully aware of the preciousness of each moment?
- Fear of planning

Underneath each of these fears is the ultimate fear that you won't be able to handle what life brings next, especially if it brings a recurrence. Thoughts of recurrence can trigger both fear and anxiety. All change provokes some level of anxiety, because it causes us to feel vulnerable. We get anxious when we are unsure of the level of risk ahead, whether the risk is to our psyches or to our bodies. Once the situation or reason for the anxiety has been addressed, the anxiety usually goes away. But when fear becomes persistent apprehension or you begin to have panic attacks, you should discuss your feelings with your doctor.

Although it might be difficult to see at first, there is a positive side to fear. Like anger, fear can be the motivator that gets you or keeps you on track. It can propel you to live a healthy life and to take better care of yourself, often for the first time. Fear of regret — of not living fully — can push you to pursue the dream you once had or encourage you to make new choices, be it a new relationship, a new job, or new leisure or travel opportunities. For some survivors, fear of recurrence provides the positive stimulus they need to clean up their lives.

> *"I have not stopped being fearful, but I have ceased to let fear control me. I am learning to go forward despite the pounding in my heart and the little voice in my head that says 'Stop, no, turn back, you'll fail if you venture too far.'"*
>
> — Janice, 56 years old, lung cancer, 1-year survivor

 SELF SCAN QUESTIONS 12, 13 AND 14 *(see page 129)*

CANCER'S UNIQUE FEARS

There are two immobilizing fears unique to cancer survivors: the fear of recurrence and the fear of stress.

Fear of Recurrence

Every survivor we've met, even those whose cancer occurred 20 years ago, speaks of the fear of the cancer returning. Fear of recurrence or of developing a secondary cancer is one of the most difficult obstacles survivors face when picking up the pieces of their post-cancer lives. "I'm always looking over my shoulder," many say, or "I feel like I'm playing with a loaded gun." With the fear of recurrence come uncertainty and an increased sense of vulnerability.

"I was obsessed with the idea of a relapse. I would wake up during the night sweating from nightmares. At least in chemotherapy I was doing something useful, instead of worrying and waiting for the cancer to come back."
— Sharon, 48 years old, colorectal cancer, 1-year survivor

Recurrence differs from an initial diagnosis. The first time you are diagnosed with cancer, your fear centres on the unknown. The second time around, you know exactly what to expect: the exhaustion, the endless appointments, the waiting, the roller-coaster of emotions, and the difficult job of fitting cancer into your life picture ... all over again. Fear is what you feel the first time; the second time it's more like dread.

"I'm terrified of having to go through chemotherapy again. I don't know if I could go there. The pain and nausea — I don't think I could live through that experience again."
— Nick, 37 years old, testicular cancer, 2-year survivor

Fear is a natural response to a threat. After cancer, you're unsure of what to expect from your body. Every new lump, mole or sore muscle triggers panic. You're sure every headache is brain metastasis and every new blemish the beginning of a tumour. If you begin to lose weight or need more sleep, it must be a sign of recurrence. After all, cancer is unpredictable, and you can never be completely sure you're cancer free.

"I was sure my backache was bone metastasis. But then I realized the amount of stress I was under and that my body was tense and my jaw clenched all the time. The increased muscle tone contributed to my backache."
— Rachelle, 32 years old, breast cancer, 4-year survivor

Some survivors experience a newfound body awareness; for others, the inclination after cancer is to turn away from the body. Now is the time to listen. But this isn't easy, given how ambiguous the body's messages are. How do you learn to pay attention to anything unusual, to trust the warning signs and seek medical help if necessary, while also allowing for the normal aches and pains of everyday life?

While an erosion of confidence in your body after cancer is normal, the mind has an amazing ability to generate fear out of any physiological stimuli. The problem is, this fear interferes with your ability to move forward in recovery. You can't enjoy the present moment, or plan for the future, when fear lurks in the background. You can't sleep well, can't concentrate on what you want to do with the rest of your life, can't focus on your health when you anticipate cancer around every corner.

> *"Every day would be marred by my fears of the cancer returning. I would wake up in the morning, and it was the first thing I'd think of. It would disable me or at the very least impair me, and I could never allow myself to be happy or carefree because I'd always be worrying about the cancer. It became far more important than it should have, but I couldn't get it under control."*
> — Isaac, 30 years old, melanoma, 1-year survivor

The fear of recurrence is, in fact, the nagging fear of death. Either that fear sits somewhere around your toes and pops up every so often, or it's in your face most of the time. Whether it announces itself as a loud drumbeat or a dull buzz in the background, when it surfaces it is terrifying.

> *"The fear is always there. Some days it reverberates so loudly it turns my world upside-down; other days it's like white noise constantly playing."*
> — Russell, 51 years old, bladder cancer, 9-month survivor

It's common to worry about the cancer coming back, especially during the first year after treatment. Survivors agree that certain events trigger this fear to flare up: follow-up visits, your annual check-up, anniversary dates of diagnosis and treatment completion, someone else's death from cancer, an article in the paper, a birthday, or seeing someone you met during your treatment in hospital.

> *"Usually it comes around the anniversary date of my diagnosis. But it can also be brought on by something out of the blue, like a certain song on the radio that reminds me of the time I spent in treatment or whenever I see*

*or smell bananas. They were the only thing I could keep down when I was
in treatment; now they make me nauseated."*

— Yolanda, 33 years old, brain cancer, 3-year survivor

All long-term survivors report that the fear of recurrence does recede with
time — particularly once you pass the five-year mark. Gradually, the volume
starts to drop and the intensity begins to lessen. The pressures and pleasures
of daily life tend eventually to push your fear of the cancer returning to the
back of your mind.

 SELF SCAN QUESTIONS 15 AND 16 *(see page 129)*

Fear of Stress

While there is no solid research linking stress with cancer and the immune
system, many survivors believe stress was a contributing factor. Stress can be
described as the body's physiological response to any demand (real or imagined) that is placed upon it. The heart rate increases, blood pressure goes up
and the body secretes adrenaline to prepare us for action. Stress is connected
to loss and to the fear of future losses. It's a psychological response triggered
by the perception that the losses can't be stopped; hence, we generally attach
negative connotations to it. When you are faced with a problem that you
can't solve, you are under stress.

Being stressed, anxious or worried exhausts us, erodes our sense of well-
being and leaves us with diminished energy. Constant, insidious stress can create such physical symptoms as headaches, insomnia, recurrent infections, and
injuries. Survivors who believe stress caused their cancer are likely to develop
a fear of stress, and this fear can appear in different forms. You might be afraid
that if you get too stressed out the cancer will return, or that stress will
weaken your immune system. You might feel stressed about not eating well,
not getting enough sleep, not relaxing, or getting too wound up. Repeatedly,
you are admonished to avoid stress, as well as to avoid white foods, avoid alcohol, avoid staying up too late: avoid, avoid, avoid. You're so busy avoiding
everything that might cause a recurrence, you can't begin to live again.

*"All I thought about was keeping the cancer from coming back. I did every-
thing I could to stay healthy. I started a strict vegan diet, exercised six days
a week, began getting an array of immune enhancing therapies, and took
a wide array of vitamins and special teas. But after eight months I had no
social life left. I couldn't go out for dinner with friends because I couldn't
eat what was on the menu, and of course, I didn't drink. I needed eight
hours of sleep and never stayed out late. I started resenting everything in
my life. I had no life: it was all about cancer."*

— Evan, 25 years old, lymphoma, 1-year survivor

Fear of stress can influence your choices and decisions. Eager to resume her
pre-cancer life, 23-year-old Meghan returned to university following the completion of her treatments for melanoma. But, she says, "There was so much
stress I quit and started selling muffins. Now I'm stress-free but feel lousy
because I'm not accomplishing what I want. I'm frightened because I don't
know what a reasonable workload is for me."

Many of us have periods in our lives when we are overextended. We can
become overwhelmed and exhausted. It is not uncommon during such times
to give up the activities that bring us relief — yoga, painting, walks on the
beach. The cancer survivor who has been pursuing a healthy lifestyle may
panic at the thought of letting go of the very tools and activities that he or
she believes helped keep the cancer at bay.

*"I love my new job. But it takes up so much of my time that I no longer do
regular exercise or get to my karate class. Recently, I've even stopped at a
fast food outlet, which after my cancer I swore I'd never do! I'm worried
that I'll have to choose between work and health."*

— Jim, 52 years old, prostate cancer, 4-year survivor

There is also much talk in cancer circles about the importance of staying
positive, about how being hopeful and having faith in the future will help
make you well. Staying positive has become a popular motivational tool during the treatment and healing process. Having a positive attitude is not nor-
mally considered a source of stress. But some survivors end up worrying

that if they don't feel positive all the time it will be their fault if they don't get well. Many survivors speak about the pressure they experience (from themselves as well as from others) to maintain a positive attitude no matter how terrible they are feeling. Staying positive can become a performance test, and you may feel like a failure if you can't put on a happy face constantly.

> *"I found trying to maintain a positive attitude incredibly draining. You are expected to be cheerful all the time, but it isn't real. Lots of people I met in treatment had positive attitudes and a strong will to live, but they still died. I think always focusing on the positive keeps you from exploring real feelings, which for me were depression and anger."*
>
> — Rudy, 24 years old, leukemia, 7-month survivor

David Spiegel, author of *Living Beyond Limits: New Hope and Help for Facing a Life-Threatening Illness*, refers to this kind of pressure as "the prison of positive thinking:" "The last thing you need is to feel bad about feeling bad." (2) Life isn't made up solely of happy moments. In order to recover, you must give yourself permission to feel each emotion that surfaces.

Much of what we hear about stress is negative. But stress is also a positive component of normal life. Stress accompanies change and is an essential part of the transformational process. While too much stress can cause burnout, too little can cause rust-out. We need a certain quota of stress to engage in healthy living. Different levels suit different people. Positive stress helps us find ways to keep a balance between work, play, and rest.

> *"You need to get back to being involved in the everyday things like, 'Who's picking Johnny up after his baseball game?' or 'What will I buy my wife for Christmas?' It helps you to fight off those intrusive thoughts about recurrence that initially come up all the time."*
>
> — Mike, 69 years old, colorectal cancer, 2-year survivor

 SELF SCAN QUESTIONS 17, 18, 19, 20 AND 21 *(see page 129)*

THE BRIGHT SIDE

Life is a kaleidoscope of emotion, ever changing from dark to bright, dull to colourful. As a cancer survivor, you will likely feel your emotions shifting quickly and often intensely. Some days you may be troubled, even filled with despair. But the next day, you might experience a lightness of being shaded with tenderness and deep satisfaction. The Sufi poet Rumi expresses this aspect of the human condition:

> *This being human is a guest house. Every morning a new arrival.*
> *A joy, a depression, meanness, some momentary awareness comes as*
>   *an unexpected visitor.*
> *Welcome and entertain them all!*
> *Even if they're a crowd of sorrows, who violently sweep your house*
> *empty of its furniture,*
> *still treat each guest honourably.*
> *He may be clearing you out for some new delight.* (3)

Gratitude

Despite the draining emotions associated with cancer, many survivors find that getting a second chance at life helps them to reconnect with the wonders of every day. Repeatedly, survivors express a deep sense of gratitude for being alive. Even with her constant pain, 46-year-old Mary, a seven-year survivor of breast cancer, starts each day with the affirmation, "Thank you, world, for another day of life." Being thankful for what you have is not always easy after you have survived cancer. It is tempting to focus on what you have lost and thus to become resentful and angry. But daily acts of appreciation and gratitude can buffer us against the forces of fear and anxiety. Feeling fortunate to be alive enhances our appreciation for life and reawakens us to the beauty and blessings that surround us.

After cancer, many survivors speak of seeing life through a new lens. Many feel their renewed appreciation and gratitude for life bring additional positive qualities to their days and aid in their recovery process. They feel more alert, energetic and engaged with the world around them. While the intensity of this gratitude can wane with time, it is initially loud and clear for almost everyone.

> *"Some days I sit in the park and watch people pass by. The children are playing, their parents are talking, the sun is shining, and I marvel at the simple pleasure of such small everyday joys."*
> — Jeannie, 58 years old, lymphoma, 2-year survivor

Some survivors express a wish to reciprocate for the many acts of generosity they received during their experience with cancer. They feel thankful and beholden: to God, to their health care team, to family and friends, to neighbours.

> *"I cannot emphasize enough how tremendous people close to me as well as casual acquaintances continue to be. They have been patient and loving beyond all I have imagined or expected. They loved me when I could not love myself, when despair was my predominant companion. I feel overwhelming thankfulness for having them in my life."*
> — Kristin, 28 years old, breast cancer, 2-year survivor

Love

Every songwriter on the planet has described the power of love. Countless TV shows, movies and best-selling stories explore how achievement, money, and power lack meaning without love. Most people are remembered not for what they did during their lives but for how much they loved. When we love unconditionally, we fill our lives with grace and feel blessed. When we reach out in love, we extend caring, understanding, joy and hope. Love is a sentiment that has a broader connotation of commitment, respect, and unselfishness. Conversely, closing our hearts to love makes us judgmental, critical, inflexible and unforgiving.

The presence or absence of love in our lives is most often connected to our relationships. Parental love, romantic love, brotherly or sisterly love, and the love among family members or good friends are all forms of love-in-relationship. But what about your relationship with yourself? It has been said that in order to love another, we must first be able to love ourselves. A healthy sense of self includes self-love, more commonly known as self-respect. This is the capacity to forgive yourself, acknowledge your strengths, be proud of your achievements, trust in your own counsel, and ultimately give selflessly to those you care about. Many cancer survivors came to love themselves for the first time.

> *"The best advice I received is that loving yourself and accepting yourself, just as you are at this moment, is a crucial step on the road to recovery. Once I decided to embrace who I was, life seemed brighter and recovery possible."*
>
> — Juliana, 32 years old, lymphoma, 7-month survivor

After cancer, many survivors feel not only a renewed love of life but also a rekindled love for family and friends. Eager to express their gratitude and appreciation, many feel as if their hearts have actually opened, allowing them to experience love in a way they never have before.

> *"I felt this big ball of energy called love. All of a sudden people were coming out of the woodwork offering me kindness and support. I know it helped me to heal."*
>
> — Karin, 23 years old, oral cancer, 3-year survivor

Happiness

Joy sustains the spirit. It puts a spring in our step and a smile on our faces. It opens us to interaction and connection with others. We live in a serious world with serious problems, cancer being one of them. While you can't delete the bad things from your mind, you can displace them with things that delight you.

We often convince ourselves that we will be happy as soon as the house is paid off or the kids get older or we lose ten pounds. This long list implies that happiness is a particular destination and we're not there yet. But happiness is both a state of mind and a way of living. It is easy to get so caught up with our daily lives that we no longer see the larger picture of who we are or what life's about. Cancer can bring the raw truth into perspective in a way the regular stresses and strains of daily living cannot. Surviving a life-threatening illness may give your life new meaning and bring your happiness more clearly into focus.

> *"The day after my one-year anniversary, I was overcome with pure joy. I was alive! In the intensity of that moment I saw all of life with a wide-open heart and different eyes. Even the rain sounded like a song."*
> — Terrance, 44 years old, brain cancer, 18-month survivor

Happiness is more than the absence of negative feelings such as anger, fear or anxiety. The emotion of happiness is described by such words as contentment, satisfaction, pleasure, and a sense of well-being. Positive experiences such as falling in love, winning a prize, or receiving the good news that your test results show no cancer can generate acute happiness. But happiness also comes from within. It is influenced by your personality as well as your attitudes and beliefs. While the source of happiness is one of the great philosophical quandaries, what matters most to survivors is getting a second chance at life and finding their own answers.

 SELF SCAN QUESTIONS 22, 23 AND 24 *(see page 129)*

MOVING FORWARD

The poet John Milton expressed the power of our thoughts, emotions and beliefs: "The mind is its own place, and in itself can make a heaven of hell, a hell of heaven." (4) You have had cancer. You have been to a terrible dark place of fear and stress. You have been angry and resentful, perhaps depressed. But you've survived. Now is the time to focus on moving forward, to learn how to hold sadness and fear in one hand and hope and trust in the other. In Section III of this book, we will suggest ways of doing just that.

SELF SCAN NUMBER 2: ASSESSING YOUR
THOUGHTS AND EMOTIONS

Your beliefs about healing

1. How have the beliefs and experiences of others influenced your own beliefs about illness? About health? About what's possible during recovery?

2. Make a list of the people you know who've had cancer and write down what happened to them. Are you relating your recovery to theirs?

3. What level of recovery do you believe is possible for yourself?

Memory issues

4. Have you noticed any problems concentrating, focusing your attention, or coming up with words or names since treatment ended? If so, does this cause problems in your day-to-day functioning? Have you considered speaking to your oncologist about your symptoms?

Acknowledging your feelings

5. What are the predominant emotions you're feeling at this time in your life?

6. Are your emotions interfering with moving forward in your recovery? If so, how?

Getting angry

7. If anger is showing up in your life, what do you think is at the root of it?

8. Do you allow yourself to feel angry, or do your beliefs about anger tell you it is wrong to experience this emotion?

9. What are you doing to manage your anger? Do you need to seek help?

Feeling sad/Feeling depressed

10. Have you been down in the dumps, unable to shake off feeling depressed most of the day, every day, for two weeks or longer?

11. If you have noticed the signs and symptoms of depression in yourself, have you sought medical help?

Feeling afraid

12. List all the fears you're currently experiencing.

13. Which fears immobilize you? Which ones might empower you to take action?

14. What are you currently doing to address your fears?

Facing the fear of recurrence

15. Rate your current level of fear of recurrence on a scale of 0-10 (with 0 being no fear and 10 being the most fear you've ever experienced).

16. Is your fear of recurrence preventing you from moving forward in your recovery? If yes, in what ways?

Checking your stress level

17. What are your primary sources of stress? List them in descending order, from the greatest stress to the smallest. Nothing is too insignificant to include.

18. Rate your current level of stress on a scale of 0 to 10 (with 0 being no stress and 10 being the most stress you've ever experienced). Next, place a number between 0 and 10 next to each of the stressors you listed in answer to question 17.

19. In what ways do your beliefs and fears about stress affect your daily life?

20. What activities help you to reduce stress?

21. Do you need support to help manage your stress?

Giving thanks

22. How does gratitude influence your life now, as compared to before the cancer?

23. How has love been renewed in your life?

24. Have the sources of your joy (playing the piano, laughing with a friend, accomplishing a goal) changed since you had cancer?

Attentive Walking

Reconnecting with the various aspects of yourself through your daily walk will not always be easy. Your body may be tired, and lack of sleep can make the walk challenging. Your emotions also affect how you move. If your mind is racing with fear, your body might feel heavier. When anger dominates your thoughts, your pace might speed up. Acknowledge your thoughts and feelings, observe how fleeting they can be, and then gently bring your attention back to the present moment. Notice where you are and appreciate that your body is moving forward. It is as important to walk when you are frightened and tired as when you are calm and energized. *Just keep walking.*

The Five-Question Check-In

When you answer the five-question check-in, try to follow your first responses, the instinctual answers that flash into your mind. Notice which question generates the greatest welling of emotion, positive or negative. Observe your feelings as they flow through you and onto the paper, without judging them. They have much to tell you.

CHAPTER SEVEN

Why Am I Here?
Assessing Your Spirituality

"I believe we walk a path that sometimes dips downwards and sometimes rises up. Cancer brings intensity to life. It demands some form of letting go. I kept praying, asking God to help me let go of the way things used to be so I can start a new life."

— Alilya, 54 years old, lymphoma, 2-month survivor

"I understand a lot more about spirit since my cancer. For me, the real meaning of life is love and compassion. I knew this before in my head, but when I got cancer I received such an outpouring of caring and love from others, it really overwhelmed me. I now believe in my heart how important a sense of connection is."

— Kathleen, 62 years old, colorectal cancer, 7-month survivor

The human life cycle, from birth to death, is often referred to as a journey. This journey includes times of happiness and joy as well as times of suffering and loss. It can also include cancer. Having a life-threatening illness is often a catalyst for exploring life's big questions, the deep, soul-searching kind that can shake us to the core: *Who am I? What's life all about? Is there a God? Is this all there is? Is there life after death?* Such questions challenge our beliefs and cause us to reflect on what really matters to us.

It is an important aspect of healing to honour and care for your spirit. Living well with the experience of cancer might include making deeper connections with others or connecting with something larger than yourself. The Self Scan questions at the end of this chapter encourage you to notice what sustains you as you forge a path to wellness, what strengthens or diminishes your spirit, and what brings your life a sense of purpose and meaning.

In his book *Choices for Healing*, Michael Lerner describes the role of spirit in healing: "The healing process not only has a tendency to bring people closer to an appreciation of who they uniquely are and what their unique purpose is in this world. It also brings them closer to God, spirit, inner peace, connectedness, or whatever we choose to call that which is great and mysterious." (1)

Cancer can be a wake-up call to the value of life, a prod to live the life we want or believe we were meant to live in the time we have left. It is often from within the realm of spirit that we seek to derive purpose and meaning for our lives. A sense of life's purpose or meaning feeds the soul and gives us a reason to get out of bed and face the perils of everyday living. The longing for meaning is a genuine human need.

WHY ME?

Because we live in a science-driven era, we have been educated to think in terms of cause and effect. But science cannot help us answer the big questions that humanity has always struggled with. These we must answer for ourselves. The need to understand why bad things happen, to find an explanation for what caused their cancer or to create meaning from their cancer experience compels survivors to explore the questions *Why me? Why now?*

Almost every survivor has a theory about what caused his or her cancer. Some believe it happened because of something they did or didn't do. These explanations involve lifestyle choices such as excessive eating or drinking, smoking, poor food choices, too much sun exposure or too much stress. Others link their cancer to genetic defects, family history or exposure to chemical toxins or environmental pollutants. Research tells us that the causes of cancer are multi-factorial. No one knows the exact cause of his or her cancer. But for those who need a specific answer, this vague not-knowing poses a problem.

"I lived a very healthy life. If I don't know why I got cancer, what am I supposed to do to keep it from coming back?"
> — Marta, 32 years old, ovarian cancer, 2-month survivor

Whether you attribute your cancer to an act of God, a twist of fate or direct exposure to toxins, at some point you, like every survivor, will develop a rationale that helps you address the question of why. All cultures have beliefs about luck, fate and destiny. These represent attempts to address and understand the deeper mysteries of life. Many survivors can't find inner peace until they have wrestled with these existential questions.

The "why" questions may also contain an element of survivor's guilt: *Why did I live when others died?* or *Why was my treatment less horrendous than what someone else went through?* It is not uncommon when one finds safety amidst human tragedy to feel guilty or to experience empathetic suffering for those who are still caught in the nightmare. But if you have found shelter from the tornado or hurricane, it is your compassion and connection to humanity that cause you to think of those still out in the storm. Suffering has no rules.

For some survivors, struggling with the "why me?" question is not so much a search for meaning as an issue of control. When you feel out of control, it is sometimes easier to blame yourself or others than to accept that there is no ready answer for what happened. While many of us live our lives under the illusion that we are in control, cancer shatters that illusion.

The only rule about cancer is that there are no rules. Try not to get stuck demanding that the numbers add up; 1+1 does not equal 2, and 2+2 does not equal 4 when you're dealing with cancer. You can't get a logical answer to an existential question.

"It isn't supposed to happen this way. Why did my mother get cancer and die only a few months after my father? Why did I get cancer in my early thirties right after marrying the man of my dreams and having our first child? It's not fair. Why should so much bad happen in just one family? I can't get past the injustice of it all."
> — Julie, 33 years old, lymphoma, 3-month survivor

Survivors with strong faith-based beliefs, citing the phrase "Thy will be done," are often able to let these questions rest. They draw comfort and support from knowing God has a plan they are unaware of. Many others eventually come to phrase the question as "Why not me?" Lightning strikes randomly. If cancer chooses indiscriminately, no one is exempt.

> *"Ultimately, I came to understand that I was no more or less valuable than anyone else. I hadn't been singled out. It was a question without an answer, but I had to ask it and work it out for myself. I finally settled on 'What was, was and what is, is.' It was the only way for me to make peace with the whole thing."*
> — Chloe, 45 years old, leukemia, 2-year survivor

The truth is we don't understand why illness happens, why it strikes certain people or why some people get better and some do not. We may never know. Somehow you will need to bring closure to the issue and make your own peace with these questions.

 SELF SCAN QUESTION 1 *(see page 149)*

SOUL SEARCHING

The "why me?" question often leads to a process of deep soul searching in which survivors take an honest look at the meaning of their lives. *Why me?* slips effortlessly into *Why am I here? What's my purpose on this earth? What's life about?*

There is nothing like the threat of death to sharpen your focus on what's truly important in your life. Finding yourself in danger or serious trouble quickly highlights who and what really matters to you and whether or not you have been behaving accordingly. Facing illness invites serious questioning and reflecting. This is the time to remove yourself from the clamour of daily life, find a quiet place, and reflect on life's bigger questions. It's a time of solitude in which to examine your heart to determine your true beliefs and explore the meaning of spirituality in your life. This may be an unfamiliar process; it may also feel uncomfortable. There's no denying that you risk calling your previous beliefs into question.

In times of despair, many people need to reaffirm their beliefs about spirituality and the sense that all is right in the world. They need to relearn their faith in the way life unfolds. They yearn for solace and connection — with the rest of humanity and with the universe as a whole. The healing process has a tendency to bring us closer to the ways of the spirit, to forge a relationship to both mystery and the divine.

"The more I connect with spirit the more it shows up in my life. I feel more balanced when my spiritual life is in focus. It gives me a sense of inner strength and peace."
— Marianne, 56 years old, breast cancer, 3-year survivor

All of us must wrestle with the great philosophical questions, finding a way to frame them that fits with our beliefs. The search for answers can lead to additional, perhaps even tougher questions: *What do I believe in? What are my truths? What are my convictions?* While the need for answers is deeply embedded in the human psyche, it is actually the search itself that teaches us to go beyond our existing knowledge and reach for a greater understanding of our role in this lifetime.

The meaning of life differs for each of us, and it shifts with both time and experience. It may not be the universal meaning of life that's important to you, but rather the specific meaning of your life at this moment. Rainer Maria Rilke describes the questioning process beautifully:

"You are so young; you stand before beginnings. I would like to beg of you, dear friend, as well as I can, to have patience with everything that remains unsolved in your heart. Try to love the questions themselves, like locked rooms and like books written in a foreign language. Do not now look for the answers. They cannot now be given to you because you could not live them. It is a question of experiencing everything. At present you need to live the question. Perhaps you will gradually, without even noticing it, find yourself experiencing the answer, some distant day." (2)

THE SPIRITUAL CONTINUUM

The terms spirit, spirituality, and religion are often used interchangeably, but they are not the same. You can be spiritual without being religious, and you can have a strong sense of spirit without following any specific discipline or set of spiritual practices. Certainly what calls to or nurtures the spirit of one person may offer no such benefit to another. But spirit, spirituality and faith all offer us ways to search for our authentic self. Many survivors speak of wanting to live a more authentic life. They seek lasting values that will nourish, rather than diminish, their lives. As you answer the Self Scan questions at the end of this chapter, we invite you to explore what nurtures your inner self, using a continuum that differentiates the areas of spirit as follows:

Spirit / Inner Wisdom	*Spirituality*	*Religious Faith*
your essence	connection to something greater than yourself	traditional religious beliefs and practices

Spirit Is Inner Wisdom

Your inner spirit is carried within your core self. It is a private area of your life that draws upon whatever calms and inspires you. It connects you to the rest of humanity. When you experience the joy of a beautiful sunrise or a deep connection to a precious work of art, it is your spirit that is touched by the experience. Your spirit is what your heart tells you is true, even when your mind can't prove it. It is your essence, your true nature, the timeless internal force that sustains meaning and hope.

Resilience is an essential part of spirit. Many cancer survivors find a renewed faith simply in the resilience that got them through their illness. This resilience revealed strength deep within that they hadn't known they possessed, and they realize they can call on it to help them move forward in recovery.

> *"Even though my body was weak and devastated by the cancer, my heart and soul became stronger and more alive."*
>
> — Keeley, 56 years old, lymphoma, 6-month survivor

Spirit is a vital force in the healing process. It may be the richest resource we have. It gives us the courage to face life's challenges, the capacity to put events into perspective, and the ability to find peace in the midst of chaos and uncertainty. The feelings of spirit are open and spacious, transcending our physical selves and our specific issues to connect us with the greater whole. What evokes spirit is unique to each individual, but many people mention being inspired by music, walks in nature, or their own creative outlets.

In matters of spirit, we seek to find the wisdom contained in our life experiences. Consequently, survivors speak of needing to quiet themselves, to remove themselves from the noise of daily life long enough to hear the voice of their own heart.

> *"When I sit quietly for a few minutes, I feel a calm come over me and I know that my strength and resilience come from deep within. It's as if a gentle hand is holding me up."*
> — Talya, 44 years old, colon cancer, 1-year survivor

Survivors with a strong spirit trust in their inner resources. They are able to relax and go with the flow, trusting life to unfold as it will. A strong spirit allows you to trust that your core self will get you through whatever triumphs and troubles may lie ahead.

Spirituality

Spirituality is a state of being in relationship with oneself, others, nature, God or a higher being. It acknowledges the presence of a power or an intelligence that is much greater than our individual selves. This power is called by many names in many different cultures: God, the Creator, the Universal Source, Gaia, the Holy Spirit, Allah, the Goddess, Brahman, the Tao, the Divine Order and the cosmos, to name but a few.

Spirituality can be found both within faith-based religions and outside of religion. Survivors with a spiritual belief system and/or practice often experience a sense of comfort, peace of mind, an inner strength that contributes greatly to an improved quality of life. Spirituality touches something deep within us. Many cancer survivors engage in spiritual practices to further their understanding of, and connection to, the divine. Through contributing to their communities, spending time in nature or engaging in meditation, prayer, and other contemplative practices, survivors seek to connect with a greater life force and find meaning in both the rational and the irrational aspects of life.

You don't need to be religious to pray. Talking to God can calm a worried mind and bring peace to a suffering heart. "Let go and let God" is an affirmation commonly used by survivors to help them surrender to the wisdom of a force more powerful than themselves.

For many survivors, cancer becomes a spiritual journey. They seek directions to a spiritual home or to a special place of beauty or tranquility that they can identify as sacred ground.

> *"For some time since my cancer I have been exploring spirituality, but I don't relate to conventional Western religion. I've spent time in sweat lodges with medicine men, in the jungle of Peru with shamans, and on retreats in solitude in a monastery. They all bring me into direct relationship with spirit, something within that connects me with the greater power of the universe."*
>
> — Jacques, 55 years old, prostate cancer, 2-year survivor

Religious Faith

Many people seek a personal relationship with God through a traditional religious discipline or practice. Religion provides a structured way for people to take care of their souls, and it can provide solace and support during troubled times. Going to church, temple, or mosque helps believers to remain conscious of moral values and ethical behaviour while providing respite from the material world. Religion provides its members with a community of people who share the same beliefs. It also offers a connection to God through a place to worship, rituals of devotion and traditional methods of marking significant life events and milestones such as birth, marriage, and death.

The way cancer affects religious faith is different for everyone. Some survivors find their existing faith deepened or their commitment strengthened by their brush with death. People who had been floundering may come to a new level of understanding of their faith.

> *"I finally understood my faith in God. It's not a question of God being on my side; it's 'Am I on God's side?' Cancer turned my thinking around."*
> — Francesca, 36 years old, ovarian cancer, 2-year survivor

Some survivors attribute their ability to make sense of the cancer experience to their faith. They know that there's a divine plan and that they need to trust in it; if death comes to the door, they believe they will be taken care of. But some find their beliefs too rigorously tested by cancer and end up turning away from their religion. *How could a benevolent God do this to me?* they ask. *What did I do to deserve this?* Cancer has shattered their trust in God, and they are angry at Him, angry at the cancer, angry at how illness has changed their lives. Others choose to abandon their beliefs in search of something new.

> *"I was just a kid, just starting out in life when I got cancer. If there really is a God who is loving and caring, why would he do this to me? I see no reason to be involved with any church."*
> — Miguel, 26 years old, lymphoma, 5-year survivor

Many people simply do not believe in God or an afterlife and are comfortable without faith-based affiliations. But on the continuum between those with a strong faith and those who distrust organized religion are many people who feel lost and long to connect with a community or a tradition. Most of us need something to hold onto in times of adversity. Many non-religious survivors say that the people they observed who relied on religion seemed to handle cancer with more ease than they did. They admire the strength of those with a religious faith and their acceptance of the situation, even if they can't go there themselves.

> *"If people don't have faith, meaning, or loving support in their lives, I believe their suffering may be greater."*
> — Geoffrey, 56 years old, prostate cancer, 4-year survivor

Ultimately, faith is an individual decision. Whether you express your spirituality through practising a traditional faith, spending time in nature, appreciating art, or being a good friend, it remains that special part of you that connects with the world outside yourself — the greater universe. Each of us must discover for ourselves what we believe in and what works for us.

> *"I found this message on a commercial greeting card. I call it my Hallmark spirituality, but it helped me understand that I do have faith, without being part of a religious group: 'Faith means not having to know where you're going, in order to believe you'll get there safely.'"*
>
> — Sally, 60 years old, breast cancer, 9-year survivor

YOUR SPIRITUAL CIRCUMSTANCES

Perhaps cancer has led you to seek spirituality for the first time. Perhaps it has pushed you to the brink of spiritual crisis or caused you to renew your faith. Every survivor's experience is different, but most people find they must confront these large issues at some point.

Searching

Cancer can herald an exciting time of discovery for survivors who have never considered spirituality or religion before. A spiritual thirst has gone unquenched, and you suddenly realize you must know where you stand. You need to read, to ponder. Perhaps you desire guidance. You are embarking on a spiritual quest to understand what life is all about. You become a seeker of truth. But you also seek stability, comfort, a more fulfilling life. You want to fill an emptiness inside you that you hadn't even realized was there before the cancer.

> *"I jumped in head first. I've explored Buddhism and Christianity. I've spent time with a local pastor and a Zen monk. It's a whole new world, and I need to find what's right for me."*
>
> — Fraser, 56 years old, melanoma, 2-year survivor

Struggling

Any crisis brings you face to face with your own soul. Many survivors experience a spiritual crisis after cancer. You can feel suddenly unplugged from the sources that once nourished you; in a word, you are disconnected. Cancer can cast doubt on beliefs you've always taken for granted. Beliefs that once brought comfort may no longer reside calmly in your mind. New or different thoughts may cause uncertainty and inner turmoil. You don't know where to turn for solace or answers. If there is a God, why would He let this happen? Why do some people suffer with multiple side effects and others walk away from their cancer experience with hardly a scratch? Why do some people die despite their best efforts and a strong positive will to live?

> *"I thought I had an understanding of my spirituality and my own belief in God, but after the cancer my beliefs were shattered. I questioned everything and began to wonder if anything I'd ever thought before was true."*
> — Nina, 53 years old, lung cancer, 3-year survivor

Struggling with these issues can be frightening, distressing and exhausting. You feel isolated, and it's as if you have lost something profound. Life seems to have no purpose.

> *"I was sent to a psychiatrist, but what I really wanted was to talk to a priest. I was chasing my mortality, and I was desperate to know what my life was all about. I wasn't mentally ill; I was in a spiritual crisis. I needed help with the meaning of my life now that it might soon be over."*
> — Kerry, 49 years old, leukemia, 2-month survivor

It can take months or years to move through this period of transition and emerge feeling whole again. But the need to question and even reject your faith may be what allows you to develop a stronger, more mature faith in the end. Many survivors do clarify their beliefs and make peace with their God.

Reconnecting

Maybe spirituality is an interest you haven't thought seriously about until now. Or you've been taking your faith for granted, and you now feel a need to renew your commitment to it. Perhaps you want to take up a daily spiritual practice, such as prayer, meditation, or spiritual reading, or to start attending worship services. You may be considering seeking out a teacher or guide. You may want to strengthen a connection that you now see has been fragile all along, neglected because of life's busy-ness.

Some cancer survivors decide to go on a spiritual retreat or visit a place of great natural beauty. Others take on some form of community service or join a spiritual community of others who share their beliefs.

> *"I began visiting the Queen Charlotte Islands, home to the Haida people. I'd sit and watch the raven, the hummingbird, the squirrels. I felt such an ancient connection there with nature and spirit."*
>
> — Anthony, 32 years old, lymphoma, 2-year survivor

 SELF SCAN QUESTIONS 2, 3, 4, 5, 6 AND 7 *(see page 149)*

MAKING PEACE WITH DEATH

We spend our lives trying to ignore, deny or outrun death. We live in fear of it. But it is the acceptance of death that leads to embracing a fuller life. After an experience with cancer, your old illusions of immortality are shaken, and you may feel robbed of the youthful invincibility and innocence that once protected you. But in their place come a new awareness and understanding.

Some cancer survivors acknowledge the threat to their existence only briefly and then quickly move on. Others explore more deeply the meaning of death.

> *"The new me is definitely more aware of mortality and more conscious of the risk of premature death. This gives me a greater appreciation of life. I try harder to live in the present instead of the future. On the down side,*

I can become more anxious about any perceived threat to my health and well being. I don't think I'm afraid of dying; it's just that I so much want to live."
— Katarina, 22 years old, osteosarcoma, 6-month survivor

Cancer catches most people by surprise; they never imagine it will happen to them. Many have never thought seriously about death before. Some survivors react by denying their mortality, preferring to pretend life hasn't changed. But others find the threat of death forces them to consider how they really want to live. The act of confronting your own death can actually help you accept your mortality and, ultimately, diminish your fear of dying.

"Maybe I'm just kidding myself when I say I'm not afraid to die, but I really feel more accepting of the life and death cycle. I met a number of people in treatment who talked about dying, even what kind of service they wanted, and some did die. You can't have cancer and not at some point think about dying."
— Bruce, 58 years old, leukemia, 6-year survivor

Being so close to death also may cause people to reassess their beliefs about what happens after you die. Even those of us with a strong faith often relegate God to church services or big religious holidays. But when death comes into your life, your relationship — or lack of one — to God takes on a whole new meaning.

"My faith was always in the background, but once I got cancer it came to the foreground very quickly. I relied more on my faith than I ever had before. It sustained me when I thought of dying."
— Stephan, 44 years old, throat cancer, 2-month survivor

Cancer also makes you think differently about time. For some, it brings a sense of urgency to the unfinished business in their lives. You may need to think about past painful events in order to see what still needs healing. While it is difficult to forgive yourself and others, forgiveness can play a big part in your ability to make peace with death.

Many survivors feel pressured to put such life-and-death issues on the back burner once their treatment has ended. They want to resume normal activities because they have already taken so much time from others in fighting the cancer. Some feel they don't have the right to take more time. But others see their brush with death as giving them the very permission they need to use their time differently — whether to address certain life lessons or to live in gratitude and appreciation for what they have.

> *"When you are faced with the prospect of dying, then living becomes more real to you. Now I take time to stop and smell the roses, and 'Carpe Diem' is my motto. My brush with death made me realize I was rushing too fast through life. I wasn't taking enough time to enjoy the people I loved or to appreciate the little gifts that every day brings."*
>
> — Bud, 55 years old, prostate cancer, 1-year survivor

You need to work through your feelings about mortality at your own pace. Some survivors confront these issues head-on; others go slowly, dipping a toe into the waters to see what happens. Others never dare to go there at all.

 SELF SCAN QUESTIONS 8, 9 AND 10 *(see page 149)*

GRIEF: OUR RESPONSE TO LOSS

Cancer reminds us how fragile life is and how vulnerable we are. Life brings many losses. These vary in intensity, but all of them give rise to grief in some form.

> *"After treatment, I felt stripped of all the layers that had made me who I was. You try to move on with the rest of your life, but you are really not the same person you once were. In some ways you are blessed with feeling more, seeing more clearly, and being more compassionate. But I believe you still have to grieve the loss of the old you."*
>
> — Pamela, 50 years old, ovarian cancer, 6-year survivor

Any significant loss affects your sense of self, and cancer brings an armful of them. Your loss might be physical: a body part or an ability. You might have lost your income, your job, a relationship, or a favourite pastime. There are also the more intangible losses, of security, of innocence, of trust in your body, of your hopes and dreams. Taken together, these losses can be overwhelming.

> *"I was going to art school before the cancer, and now I can't go back because I've lost part of my arm and don't want to be around so many toxic fumes and dangerous chemicals. It's not only that I have to change my profession, but I have to give up my dream of being an artist."*
> — Alex, 20 years old, osteosarcoma, 8-month survivor

The only way through loss is grief. We need to grieve our losses — to honour and process our sadness and distress — in order to recover and move forward. As difficult and unfamiliar as the feelings may be, grieving helps you make the transition from post-treatment cancer to living well. It involves sorting through the challenges and changes you've experienced, deciding what to hang onto and what to let go of. It means telling your cancer story over and over again — as many times as you need to — in order to feel the healing medicine that happens in the telling as well as in knowing you have been heard by others. Each retelling reveals new insights, uncovers hidden emotions and allows your story to unfold as it should from here.

In the early days after treatment ends, grief may seem like a distant land. You may still be trying to process what just happened. The sadness over the magnitude of your loss may seem unbearable. You may be stunned, disoriented or depressed. Your new reality may be too unsettling right now. But with each passing day comes the ability to live with the changes and limitations, and the new you begins to emerge from the fog.

Moving forward doesn't necessarily mean that grieving ends. Medical social worker Lis Smith states, "Our society does not allow people to grieve long enough. Your partner of 35 years dies, and it is not long before others expect you to be done with grieving and put it away on the shelf. I don't believe grief stops; I believe it just changes its intensity and shape with time." (3)

Grieving challenges you to relinquish some part of yourself, even before you are sure what will replace it. You must trust that you will survive the loss in order to move on.

As you grieve, it is natural for sorrow to give way at times to anger, even rage. Your way of life, your beliefs, your confidence in who or what you can trust have all been shaken. Although the future was always unknown and uncertain, you now know on a deeper, more personal level what that means. There is a new tension between healing and living and loss.

Cancer can also be the catalyst for dealing with the grief associated with unresolved issues in your life — a parent or child's death, the loss of a job, a divorce, or previous physical or emotional traumas. Past losses are sure to surface in times of crisis, especially if they had been ignored or denied.

> *"While dealing with the loss and grief associated with my own diagnosis and side effects, I came to know exactly how my mother must have felt when she was diagnosed years before. I hadn't understood at the time and now I feel even worse that I hadn't been there to support her. I had a lot of unresolved grief that I didn't even know was there until I was diagnosed with cancer."*
>
> — Hardeep, 39 years old, breast cancer, 2-year survivor

How you grieve is highly personal. The intensity of the pain and the length of the grieving process will vary from person to person. Both are influenced by our previous experiences with loss and by our cultural, philosophical and religious beliefs. Slowly, though, you will find your way into a new life.

This is only the briefest introduction to grieving. There are many excellent books on the subject, and we recommend some of them in the resource section at the end of this book. It is also important to get whatever support you need as you move through the grieving process, be it from friends, family, support groups, a faith community or professional counselling.

 SELF SCAN QUESTIONS 11, 12, 13 AND 14 *(see page 149)*

HOPE

While the stories of cancer survivors are filled with fear and anxiety, there is always hope. It is with renewed hope that survivors return home after treatment to resume their lives. Hope is desire and expectation rolled into one. It is the entry point to our hearts' yearnings. When we hope, we call upon a faith that everything will turn out well, or that it will all make sense, even if the end result is not one we chose.

We need to protect our hopes at the times it seems nothing or no one in the world supports them. The loss of hope leaves us feeling defeated and unsure of how to proceed. When you lose hope in the future, life feels dark. Without hope you live in disbelief and fear, both of which lead to feeling a loss of control. Hope can be your life preserver. It is the attitude that buoys you in the sea of transition when side effects or fears threaten to sink you.

Hope is always possible, even in the direst of circumstances. No matter what your diagnosis, no matter the statistics that seem to be against you, where there is life there is hope. You've made it this far; who can dare to tell you that you won't make it farther? Your core self has shown you that you have what it takes to survive; why shouldn't you thrive? Perhaps your hope is a mere sliver of light in the darkness. "Only a small crack," wrote Alexander Solzhenitsyn, "but cracks make caves collapse." (4)

Most of us have never thought much about the role hope plays in our lives. Yet many survivors report that it was hope that got them through treatment. They expected to recover and had a strong desire to do so. They hope now to live well after the cancer experience, they hope for a long life, and they hope for strength should the cancer return. Having hope helps people endure physical trauma, emotional pain, spiritual challenges, and relationship conflicts.

"I never lost hope that one day I'd be able to go back to school and do all those normal things like get a job, do some volunteer work, and return to the sports I love."

— Brianna, 25 years old, lymphoma, 5-year survivor

In the face of suffering, hope helps us find meaning and purpose. We use phrases like *Hope springs eternal*, *I hoped and prayed*, and *I'm not worried, I'm hopeful* to encourage ourselves onward in the face of adversity. Hope is our antidote to fear. It is in the hope that things can improve that we set goals and take action. Our actions engage us with life, thereby rekindling hope, which in turn propels us into the future. Hope resides within the core self and is an essential source of inspiration for moving through the transition from survivor to living well.

An important component to your recovery is that you pursue your hopes. To do this, you will need to be clear about what your hopes are.

 SELF SCAN QUESTIONS 15, 16 AND 17 *(see page 150)*

HONOURING THE SPIRIT

Often the greatest source of hope is some form of spirituality. Many survivors eventually come to appreciate spirit and faith as essential components of their lives. Without them, you may feel as if you are merely going through the motions of life, existing without passion or zest.

The ultimate goal of spirituality is a connection to others and to a higher power that transcends suffering, gives life meaning and allows you to live well. Cancer may make this connection more necessary, but it also provides the impetus you need to get there.

SELF SCAN NUMBER 3: ASSESSING YOUR SPIRITUALITY

Asking life's big questions

1. Have you asked the "why me?" and "why now?" questions? If so, have you been able to make peace with them and lay them to rest within your belief system?

Finding sustenance and connection

2. Where do you draw your strength from in times of crisis?
3. What role does spiritual belief or religious faith have in your life?
4. In what ways has cancer affected your beliefs or faith?
5. Do you create times of quiet contemplation for yourself? What happens during those times?
6. How has your connection to your community or to nature changed since having cancer?
7. What ignites your inner spirit?

Facing mortality

8. What are your beliefs about death?
9. How do your beliefs and fears about death influence how you currently live your life?
10. What gives your life meaning, especially when you're feeling down or afraid? Has this changed since you've had cancer?

Experiencing grief

11. List the tangible and intangible losses you've experienced since your cancer experience.
12. Have any old feelings of loss or grief resurfaced since your cancer experience? If so, do you tend to ignore these or to address them as they arise?
13. How do you grieve?
14. Do you feel as if you need help in managing your grief?

Finding hope

15. What do you hope for in relation to your recovery and health?
16. What gives you hope?
17. What takes your hope away?

CHAPTER EIGHT

Who Showed Up?
Assessing Your Relationships

"My husband and kids just wanted the old me back. Their attitude was, 'It's over, you beat it, hey, what's for dinner?' But it was definitely not over for me. I was no longer the person I had been before. For one thing, I was tired all the time, and I couldn't do many of the activities I used to do. But there were also positive changes happening internally, and this was a welcome change. I am glad I'm not the old Laurie. I like who I am now. I just want to get better and go forward. But the reality is, even if I feel like a different person, I still have to figure out what's for dinner."

— Laurie, 48 years old, breast cancer, 3-year survivor

"Cancer does one of two things to a relationship: it either brings you closer together, or it tears you apart. Maybe it was just a case of exhaustion; we had spent so much energy fighting the illness and getting through all of the hard parts, but in the end it left us numb. The cancer split us. It was hard for my wife to understand why I didn't have any emotional where-withal left. I was exhausted; I was a changed man."

— David, 37 years old, brain cancer, 1-year survivor

When a crisis happens to someone we care about, it affects us as well. We worry, lose sleep and try to show love and support while grappling with our own fears. Cancer changes you. It will also change your relationships.

After treatment, both you and those close to you are in transition. It is an uncomfortable time, uncertain and stressful. You're feeling tired and vulnerable; so are they. You faced your own mortality; they had to face the thought of losing you. Everyone's emotions are heightened, and no one is sure what to expect next.

Supportive family members and understanding friends can be of invaluable help as you sort through the many changes brought about by cancer. But sometimes your partner or good friends can let you down. Survivors frequently report how angry and disappointed they are with people they had anticipated would be there for them but were not. In contrast, they also express surprise and gratitude towards those who did show up, many of them people whose help they had never expected. Many cancer survivors come to know love at a far deeper level, and this brings them tremendous joy and appreciation for others.

> *"I cannot say enough about the huge role my husband and close friends have had in my healing process. They continued to be patient with me long after treatments stopped, and gave me permission to talk about all feelings — especially fear — even though it was difficult for them. I never felt as though my feelings were dismissed or glossed over. They loved me when I could not love myself, when despair was my predominant companion and I was not much fun to be around."*
>
> — Eileen, 61 years old, colon, 3-year survivor

The questions in the Self Scan at the end of this chapter ask you to look at the many roles you play in the relationships in your life and at the expectations that surround these roles. In answering these questions you will first explore your relationship with yourself, then move to clarifying the impact that other key relationships have on both your life and the healing process.

ROLES AND EXPECTATIONS

Every relationship carries its own roles and expectations. Healthy relationships replenish our physical, emotional and spiritual energy. Unhealthy ones

consume and deplete us. We have expectations both of others and of ourselves, and others in turn expect certain things of us. While you are fighting
the battle with cancer, roles are often suspended or reversed. People rise to
the occasion, help out and assume your responsibilities. But after treatment
is over, they expect you to resume your old roles, sometimes long before
you're ready.

> *"My husband went non-stop doing the shopping, cooking, and laundry,*
> *along with his job, as I was literally wiped out from the chemotherapy and*
> *radiation. Our roles changed dramatically, and it was hard on the relation-*
> *ship, because I wanted to help and felt like a burden because I couldn't.*
> *However, now he wants to resume his old life ASAP, but I still need him*
> *to keep helping with at least some of these tasks for a little longer, while*
> *I build up my strength and sort through my thoughts."*
> — Sandra, 37 years old, lymphoma, 6-month survivor

> *"My sister said to me, 'Now it's your turn to take care of our parents.'*
> *At home I'm a wife, mother, and daughter-in-law. At work, I wear many*
> *hats. I'm always tired and still have some pain, but most of all my head*
> *is whirling with emotions. I'm overwhelmed with what everyone expects*
> *of me."*
> — Asya, 46 years old, breast cancer, 2-month survivor

Family beliefs and cultural values both affect how people see their roles.
Taking time to heal can be perceived in some families as taking time off. At
the other extreme, family members may see you as too fragile to resume
activities that you are eager to begin, effectively smothering you in their
attempt to care for you.

Along with changing family roles, survivors experience changing expectations at work, sometimes including incidents of discrimination or deferen-
tial treatment by co-workers. Some find that cancer has caused changes that
limit their former capabilities. Others discover their own expectations have
changed. They may decide to seek more personal fulfillment from their job,
or alternatively, come to place less importance on the workplace.

"Cancer gave me the impetus to change jobs. I realized my life was too short to give up so much time and energy to a job that drained me."
— Rabinder, 34 years old, leukemia, 2-year survivor

There are also expectations around the giving and receiving of care and attention. If your cancer has been long and difficult, your support people are likely tired. Now that you are okay, repressed emotions may surface. Feelings of anger and resentment as well as fear and depression can arise in both the survivor and his or her significant others.

A friend may feel you have not been appreciative of her efforts. Or you may feel she did not give you the love and care you needed.

Many survivors find that after cancer their roles and expectations need to be clarified. Philosophically, it is easy for family and friends to acknowledge that cancer is a life-altering experience. But on a day-to-day basis, they don't really expect to see their loved one change. After Gerrard's chemotherapy treatments were over, his family assumed he would put the cancer experience behind him and pick up where he'd left off. In reality, he was far from ready to resume his old role.

*"I didn't want to go back to my old life. I was living someone else's defini-
tion of who I was. My parents had a plan for my life, but it wasn't working
for me anymore. I was done with playing it safe. I made a 180-degree turn,
sold everything, left my job, and moved to Los Angeles."*
— Gerrard, 39 years old, lymphoma, 1-year survivor

Some survivors experience pressure to do just the opposite. Not long after her last treatment, Rhona had the unrealistic expectations of others to contend with.

*"My family asked me what mountain I'm going to climb now. After all,
Lance did the Tour de France, right? Now that I'd survived cancer, it was as
if they expected me to move on to some other great feat of heroism. I've
already climbed the mountain of cancer, and I'm trying to make sense of
what just happened to me."*
— Rhona, 37 years old, breast cancer, 4-month survivor

Because treatment can rob you of physical stamina, as a survivor you often find yourself in the position of having to ask for and accept help. If you've always been the giver of support, this adjustment may not come easily.

"I used to be a fixer in our family, not the one that needed fixing. It was a tough new role to be in."
— Angelina, 48 years old, rectal cancer, 2-year survivor

Some survivors came to realize they had been playing a particular role because they wanted to feel loved, appreciated or admired. They were the "good girl" or the "good boy," living up to everyone else's expectations, never causing a stir, always being the one everyone could count on. Cancer forced them to ask themselves what really mattered.

"I always did everything right. I was bright, dependable and cheerful. It wasn't that I wanted to change any of that; I just needed to really look at why I was doing what I was doing. Was it because I wanted to, or because I felt I had to?"
— Lindsay, 41 years old, ovarian cancer, 1-year survivor

Cancer challenges the roles we play in all aspects of our lives. Some roles we decide we are grateful for, and others we need to change. Negotiating the expectations and desires of others requires open communication and time to sort through the changes.

 SELF SCAN QUESTIONS 1, 2 AND 3 *(see page 175)*

Your Relationship with Yourself: The New You or the Old One?

Many survivors feel incredible pressure from within, as well as from others, to return to their old self, to "get back to being the Cindy we know and love." Family and friends are as surprised and unprepared as you are for the lingering side effects of fatigue, sadness or confusion. All they want is to breathe a sigh of relief, celebrate your victory over cancer, and move on.

Unfortunately, that isn't going to happen.

> *"I won't kid you. There are two Lance Armstrongs, pre-cancer and post.*
> *Everybody's favourite question is, 'How did cancer change you?' The real*
> *question is, 'How didn't it change me?' I returned a different person, liter-*
> *ally. In a way, the old me did die, and I was given a second life."*
>
> — Lance Armstrong, *It's Not about the Bike* (1)

For some survivors, knowing that life will never be the same again leads to confusion and depression. Transition can be a lonely time. You have counted on others for so much already, and you are reluctant to ask for more support. So you tuck in your fears and concerns, which only adds to your isolation. In any case, no one wants to believe there is anything wrong. Your treatments are over, you're a survivor. Case closed.

> *"I couldn't believe when a friend said to me, 'You look so well, you couldn't*
> *have had a very bad case of cancer.' She made me feel as if the cancer was*
> *no big deal."*
>
> — Rachel, 53 years old, breast cancer, 2-year survivor

Whether your sense of self is undergoing a major renovation or a minor rearrangement, cancer knocks the wind out of you. As you come to terms with the new you — your new feelings and insights, as well as any new physical limitations — it is time to examine what you can fairly expect of yourself.

> *"I was 59 years old, a healthy and active family man running my own med-*
> *ical practice, when I was diagnosed with prostate cancer. I had a poor prog-*
> *nosis, but I didn't believe it. I thought I'd go through treatment and then*
> *just get on with my life again; after all, there are well-established treat-*
> *ment protocols for prostate cancer. I was more worried about how my wife*
> *and daughters would take the news. So I waited for a few weeks before I*
> *even told my wife, and I never did tell my daughters.*
>
> *"Once treatment began, everything changed. In a few short hours, I*
> *was transformed from a hard-working doctor into a patient. But that was*

*only the beginning of the changes that would strip away the layers of who
I was. I came out of the treatment incontinent and impotent. I didn't want
to wear a diaper, so I was afraid to go out, afraid to go back to work, even
afraid to laugh.*

*"My fears and my sexual dysfunction began affecting my relation-
ship with my wife. I was no longer a patient, nor was I back to being the
strong, decisive doctor she had married. Neither she nor I had any idea
what was happening or how to find our way back to our old life together.
We both had to accept, however reluctantly, just how different I was after
cancer, both physically and emotionally."*

— Ted, 59 years old, prostate cancer, 9-month survivor

Living with cancer is a process of integration, a weaving together of your
pre- and post-cancer selves, a movement from patient to survivor, from sick
to healthy, from survivor to living well. The ultimate goal is wholeness. But
as you begin this redefinition of yourself, you may find yourself questioning
your very identity. It's as if your former self were still there, waving to you
from another time, but you're not sure you want to wave back. It's a true
paradox that you can both be yourself and someone new. The perspective is
dizzying. At times you will feel like shouting *Will the real me please stand up?*

Cancer has a way of invading your sense of self, of taking over and
pushing you aside.

*"I used to feel like somebody, until I went into the hospital where they poke
and prod and you have to wear an ugly, flimsy green gown. I felt stripped
of my identity as a mother, wife, journalist, and lover; now I was only a
patient. Once treatment finished I was labelled a survivor. I didn't know
what to make of this new identity. What does it mean to be a survivor?"*

— Veronica, 51 years old, cervical cancer, 4-month survivor

During treatment, many survivors held tight to their core sense of who they
were so as to not become the illness. They did not want the cancer to define
them. It had already taken enough. Now the label of "survivor" may feel too
fragile, too insignificant. While you are no longer suffering from the disease,

you are still learning to cope with its many side effects.

For many survivors, the redefinition of identity is a process that moves through several stages. You will need time to adapt to each new phase, making sure you feel comfortable in each one before moving on. Eventually you will come to a place that defies labelling. You'll come to rest with your inner strength, your essence. This is who you are. It took Isabelle five years to reach that point.

> *"The first three years I'd say, 'I am a breast cancer survivor.' The fourth year I heard myself say, 'I am a woman with breast cancer.' Finally I came to realize I was a woman who was active and healthy and living a full life. I didn't include the breast cancer in my description any longer."*
>
> — Isabelle, 49 years old, breast cancer, 5-year survivor

Some survivors repeat a phrase such as "very slowly" to remind themselves that healing happens in its own time. The road to a new life is long and often requires years of travel. "Know thyself" may become your new mantra.

> *"Gradually I woke up to how I was treating myself and others. I was abusing my body. I was wrapped up in jealousy and envious of everyone else. There was a lot of negativity in my life. I was mad at my husband, short-tempered with my children and not a very good friend. I decided to change it all. I let it all go and began anew."*
>
> — Lillian, 47 years old, cervical cancer, 9-month survivor

Adjusting to all the changes can leave you in a state of disequilibrium. Anxiety about your current and future capabilities is bound to generate strong emotions such as blame, guilt, anger, loss of confidence and self-esteem.

> *"I've lost my way. Ever since treatment, my excitement for life is gone. I lost a few friends and made several family members angry. I spent my life savings because I thought I was going to die. Now all I have left is a shattered life."*
>
> — Andrew, 41 years old, melanoma, 4-month survivor

At other times, you may feel a renewed appreciation for life. You may relish this new post-cancer you, finding joy in simple daily pleasures. Some survivors describe this as falling back in love with life. Many survivors divide their lives into two parts — before the cancer and after — as if drawing a line in the sand.

> *"Before cancer, I was very detail-oriented, slow, and methodical; I weighed all the options. After cancer I'm more spontaneous. I have a go-for-it attitude, and although I don't rush stupidly into things, I don't hesitate to act on an impulse. My post-cancer life has more fun and laughter in it."*
> — Luca, 33 years old, testicular cancer, 7-year survivor

Our world functions on facts, logic and practical action. But recovering your sense of self means learning to trust your intuition, insights and inner wisdom. This begins with your relationship with yourself — your self-awareness and ultimately your self-acceptance.

> *"I decided to get real with myself — look at my life, make changes, be honest with what I was feeling. It was the first time I had ever stopped to look. It was a hard place to be in, but I wanted to emerge from this experience headed in the right direction. I changed my life in so many ways. I started a new diet, stopped drinking, started exercising, and I lost weight. I began mending relationships that had gone sour. I'm gentler with the dog. I cuddle on the couch with my wife. For the first time, I'm singing around the house."*
> — Jonathon, 63 years old, prostate cancer, 2-year survivor

While it is true you will not feel the same after cancer as you did before, it is also true that you will, eventually, feel normal again. But remember, normal is not a constant in our lives: it is a state that is continually shifting in response to the unending changes we experience.

> *"Maybe life doesn't have to get back to normal, and maybe normal wasn't all that great to begin with."*
> — Reggie, 59 years old, lung cancer, 3-month survivor

Regardless of whether your process is as simple as asking yourself a few key questions or involves a longer, more gradual transformation, regaining a sense of self depends on acknowledging the changes happening to you, within you, and around you since your cancer.

 SELF SCAN QUESTIONS 4 AND 5 *(see page 175)*

Your Relationship with Your Partner: What about Us?

When cancer intrudes on your life, your relationships respond and shift. A life-threatening illness strips away illusions and challenges the status quo for both you and your partner.

> *"I always say, 'We had cancer,' because although my wife physically had the cancer, it changed our whole family. When you go through cancer with someone you love, you change just as much as they do."*
>
> — David, 43 years old, husband of Sarah,
> 3-year survivor of colon cancer

Cancer tests your relationship with your partner or spouse. It can provide an opportunity for the two of you to deepen your love. It can also be the thing that splits you apart. You and your partner both must deal with fear and uncertainty. Your partner may have been and could still be afraid of losing you. He or she no doubt felt powerless watching you suffer during treatment. You partner may well have tried to protect you by not expressing fears or by staying strong to keep things from falling apart. You may have felt supported by that, or you may have found your partner's unwillingness to talk about feelings difficult, even insensitive.

Once the physical battle with cancer is over, the psychological struggle intensifies. Even when couples have the same feelings, misunderstanding and poor communication can get in the way of being able to console each other. Here is an example: She says: *He tells me he hears me, but he really doesn't listen. Whenever I want to talk about my fears, he looks away and doesn't want to go there.*

He says: *She starts to tell me about her fears and it tears me up. I don't want her to see me scared. She needs me to be strong.*

Survivors continue to need support from others long after treatment ends. Couples require time and sometimes professional help to work through their emotions and find their way back to each other. After the drama of treatment ends, you and your partner may need to rebuild your feelings of connection and intimacy. It is important to understand that your feelings are normal, and also that your partner may not be able to meet all of your emotional needs. Everybody has limits. Figure out what you can get from him or her and then take the initiative to get the additional support you need from friends, other family members, a counsellor, a support group or your spiritual community.

> "Within a year of recovery, my partner and I started having marital difficulties. I think she couldn't cope with the person I had become. She had supported me — was like a saint all through treatment — but after the treatment she was really expecting things to go back to the way they were before the cancer. The problem is I'm different now, and all is not well in paradise."
>
> — Brian, 45-years-old, melanoma, 2-year survivor

When cancer causes you to reorder your priorities or change your outlook on life, your partner may feel left behind. Perhaps you no longer share the dreams the two of you once held for the future. Mike, 37 years old and a six-month survivor of lung cancer, felt it urgent to live life to the fullest, which included travel and new creative experiences. He wanted to spend everything — time and money — and he wanted his wife to be with him. She, however, wanted to pay off their mortgage and save for their future. While they very much wanted to be together, after cancer it felt as if they were no longer on the same page. Mike wasn't sure how much time he had left, and he became frustrated and angry when his wife refused to see things the way he did. It wasn't until after the five-year mark that he believed strongly enough in his future to make long-term plans again.

Often the differences that develop in a relationship are more attitudinal.

46-year-old Kyle, a one-year survivor of lymphoma, developed a "don't sweat the small stuff" attitude that drove his partner crazy. He wanted to relax and not worry about such mundane things as the dirty dishes piling up in the sink. His wife became more fastidious, obsessively cleaning and trying to put everything back in order. She was in a hurry to return to the life they had shared before cancer.

In Chapter Five, we reviewed some of the sexual problems survivors might experience following surgery, chemotherapy or radiation treatments. In the early days after treatment, many survivors report feeling like strangers in their own bodies. Fatigue, pain, and a lack of emotional connection, along with a range of other difficult emotions, can disrupt physical intimacy, which is bound to alter a relationship. Feelings of fear and doubt are normal on both sides. Your partner is relieved that your treatment is over but unsure of how to proceed. Each of you must find a way to communicate your needs. Most couples require patience, acceptance and time to rebuild the trust and intimacy they once shared.

> *"Though my husband says he still finds me attractive, I wonder if it's true. He's been so incredible through the whole thing, but I am never going to show him my stoma. We've always had a very open and comfortable relationship, but I am not going to share this new part of myself with him. When he comes into the bathroom or bedroom, I hide myself."*
>
> — Camille, 42 years old, colorectal cancer, 8-month survivor

Some relationships grow stronger after cancer. The two of you may feel united by your fight against a disease that threatened to tear you apart. You may experience a newfound tenderness for each other. Some people laugh more. Others dance more often. Both partners may respond to the wake-up call and develop a "seize the day" attitude, selling everything to travel the world or joining a volunteer organization in a developing country. Some couples make lists of ten things to do before they die and get busy ticking them off. The two of you could learn how to sky dive, take flying lessons or buy a boat and sail the South Pacific.

Some relationships also end — that's the reality. The pressure can become too much to bear, and difficulties that existed before the cancer experience may be intensified. Maybe your partner leaves during your treatment or shortly after. Sometimes a partner leaves during recovery, unable to cope with who the survivor has become. Abandonment at this crucial time in your life becomes another wound for you to heal from. Some survivors even find break-up more difficult than the cancer. And sometimes you will be the one who decides to leave: fear of a shortened life or disappointment in your partner's reaction to your cancer may prod you to end a relationship that isn't working.

"We never saw eye to eye after I was diagnosed with cancer. He couldn't cope with the fact that I was different, physically and mentally. We grew distant and eventually we split. When I look back I can see that it was coming; cancer was just the last straw."

— Molly, 45 years old, breast cancer, 3-year survivor

There is yet another side to the prismatic effect cancer has on primary relationships, which involves both guilt and gratitude. Paul, newly married at the time he was diagnosed, explains:

"I felt tremendously guilty and sad knowing what my wife had to go through. It was harder for her. I didn't have a choice — I had to sit there and take the treatment — but she did. She could have said, 'I'm not going through this with you, I'm not going to the hospital every day, I'm not cleaning up your vomit after chemotherapy,' but she did it all and more. How can I ever repay her? I want to make our life better because she helped me through this ordeal."

— Paul, 28 years old, lymphoma, 18-month survivor

Relationships are complicated, and cancer only adds to the complication. Every couple will cope with the experience in their own way.

 SELF SCAN QUESTIONS 6 AND 7 *(see page 175)*

Your Relationship with Your Family: A Group Experience

Cancer puts enormous stress on the family unit. During an illness, a family reveals its truths, beliefs and strengths. Once you finish treatment and the celebrations are over, your loyal supporters are eager for life to get back to normal. But survivors and their family members agree that the recovery period can be as troublesome and disturbing as treatment. Everyone is tired. Fears of mortality remain at the surface. No one is quite sure how to treat you, and they may continue to approach you with kid gloves. Or perhaps people are tired of the special treatment you have received and have begun to respond with impatience, resentment and even anger to the amount of time recovery is taking.

> *"Once I got home I didn't want to be treated like a patient anymore. I'm not an invalid. I want to heal, but I get the feeling no one knows what to do with me. I can't stand the sympathy. I just want things to be the way they were."*
>
> — Lowell, 22 years old, melanoma, 3-month survivor

In their book *Cancervive*, Susan Nessim and Judith Ellis talk about the need to allow everyone in the family their own time to process what has happened: "Cancer emotionally pressurizes the entire family. An essential part of the recovery period involves allowing everyone to decompress at a rate and in a way that is comfortable for each person." (2)

Often both survivors and their families are surprised by the intensity of the disturbances resulting from cancer. Whether the family dynamics prior to the diagnosis were healthy or dysfunctional, cancer changes the rules for everyone. In some families people avoid talking about cancer and withdraw from the survivor in subtle or obvious ways. In other families everyone plays the cheerleader, always upbeat and happy. Survivors may try to protect their family from further anguish by playing along.

> *"I'm not telling my husband or children how hard things still are for me or how I truly feel. I don't want them to worry about me. They've worried enough already."*
>
> — Angela, 42 years old, breast cancer, 6-month survivor

But protecting the feelings of others at the expense of your own may mean you won't get the help and support you genuinely need. It can also cause difficulties later on, when loved ones discover you have not been honest. In families where everyone is discouraged from expressing their feelings, recovery can be a lonely and isolating experience.

> *"Everyone is scared to say the wrong thing. So all I hear is, 'You're okay, you'll be fine.' I know they're just trying to be positive, but it shuts me down. I want to be able to tell them how I really feel."*
> — Brenda, 25 years old, cervical cancer, 2-month survivor

Some cancer survivors worry about the genetic or hereditary link within families: will cancer strike their children or siblings too?

> *"By getting cancer, I was letting 'The Side' down. I didn't want to be the one to bring this dreaded disease into my family."*
> — Donna, 47 years old, breast cancer, 4-month survivor

Issues that existed in your family before cancer will usually be waiting for you once your treatments are over. Long-standing difficulties aren't likely to be resolved during times of crisis. Past disappointments can resurface, and if family members were unsupportive or let you down during treatment, you can't expect those feelings to just go away.

> *"My brother was physically and emotionally absent when my mom was sick and then when I was sick. I haven't forgiven him for that. He could have shown up, been a part of our lives, but he chose not to."*
> — Erica, 37 years old, leukemia, 2-year survivor

Thankfully, cancer can also provide a family with the opportunity to heal old wounds and emerge united. It takes a strong resolve and sometimes outside support, but the risk and effort are worth the outcome. Some survivors experience reconciliations with family members they've been out of touch with for years. Some people begin to express their feelings for each other only after illness has threatened to take one of them away. In some situations, cancer becomes the impetus for transformation.

> *"We were a family that never talked about illness. At one point in my treatment I said to my dad, 'I love you.' We never say that in our family. He said, 'I love you, too.' That was a big step for him. I thought, 'That's all I need right now.'"*
>
> — Jory, 29 years old, head/neck cancer, 1-year survivor

Cancer changes the family climate, and each family member must be allowed to deal with the impact of cancer in his or her own way. It's a fine balance, but eventually life will settle into a new rhythm.

 SELF SCAN QUESTIONS 8 AND 9 *(see page 175)*

Children: A Special Case

The unique relationship between a parent and child is particularly taxed by cancer. Children experience the same emotions that adults do, including fear, dread, anger, and resentment. They want the cancer to be over, and they need reassurance that their parent is safe.

Studies on the impact of a parent's cancer on children show that the most important things you can do are to communicate with your children in an age-appropriate way and to disrupt their usual schedules as little as possible. Younger children need to be reassured that someone will always be there to take care of them. Adult children want you to be honest about your feelings and want to know the prognosis.

While some children will cling tighter to a parent diagnosed with cancer, others may want to ignore that cancer exists. It is not uncommon for a child to withdraw from a parent who is ill, and feelings of rejection can leave both parties feeling isolated and hurt.

> *"One of the hardest parts of my recovery involved my relationship with my son. He was three, and a special needs child. We were extremely close, but*

during and after the treatments I couldn't pick him up. For several weeks I couldn't hold him, and he couldn't understand that. He started to withdraw from me. Even though I understood he was protecting himself, it was heartbreaking for me."

— Cobe, 49 years old, brain cancer, 1-year survivor

An older child may seek support from outside the family unit. Often friends from school or outside activities fill a need that the family can't, but it can be hard for a child or young adult to find the right person to talk to.

"My daughter was at university at the time and involved with volleyball, so she had very little time to be with me. She went into a deep depression because she thought she was losing her mother. I am a single mother; she has no other relatives around. I was struggling with recovery, and the only kids she knew were these young women on the volleyball team. Talking about cancer was the furthest thing from their minds."

— Sarah, 58 years old, ovarian cancer, 4-year survivor

For some children, the reality is that their lives will become more difficult because of the cancer. They are included in the role reversal process and may be needed to help pick up the slack when one parent is too ill to participate in family tasks. Resentment and anger can result as time moves on and previous roles aren't resumed as quickly as everyone had hoped.

"My husband was the buffer between the kids and me. He wanted me just to focus on taking care of myself, and my daughter, who was fourteen, bore the brunt of a lot of additional demands, which I didn't realize at the time. Now, even at 30, she is still bitter that she 'lost her teenage years' to my cancer."

— Sylvie, 61 years old, oral cancer, 16-year survivor

Children are afraid when a parent gets sick. Though your instinct is to protect your children from difficult emotions, their fears need to be addressed. Full communication can stave off hours of imaginary horrors the child might otherwise experience. Often it's years later before your child decides to tell you how he or she was really feeling.

> *"My son, who was fourteen years old when I was diagnosed, used to run home after school every day to make sure I was still alive. I didn't know this until sometime later. It was a heart-wrenching thing to hear that he was going through such anguish. He still wants to be home after school to see if I'm okay. You try to make sure your children are not unduly frightened; at the same time you need to let them know what the deal is. It's a tightrope you're walking."*
>
> — Evelyn, 47 years old, breast cancer, 5-year survivor

Cancer has a big impact on everyone in the family, but parents can take heart from the fact that children are remarkably resilient and often wise beyond their years. Just like you, they can work their way through this difficult time.

> *"After it was all over I asked my daughter, who is sixteen and had always been very close to me, if she was still afraid that I was going to die. She said, 'Now you're a survivor of cancer, Mom, so we're all survivors with you.'"*
>
> — Francine, 45 years old, melanoma, 1-year survivor

 SELF SCAN QUESTIONS 10 AND 11 *(see page 175)*

Your Relationships with Your Friends: Who Stood by You?

Survivors often come through treatment with a different understanding of their friendships. There can be great joy over deepening friendships and heartbreak over the friendships that are lost. Along with noting the support they received from people they would never have expected to be there, almost all survivors have stories of a few friends who didn't come through for them. Sometimes this happens with a close friend, someone you have known for years.

> *"I had a girlfriend who has had a lot of troubles for years, and I've always been there for her, being reassuring and very supportive. But when I had*

cancer, she was actually a little annoyed that I didn't have the energy to give her my support anymore. She stopped calling, and I felt very disappointed she couldn't be there for me."

— Melissa, 28 years old, thyroid cancer, 3-month survivor

As you already know, friends react in different ways to a diagnosis of cancer. Some come forward right away with unending support. Others show up awkwardly and don't know what to say or do. You will likely also have some friends who simply cannot deal with your cancer; you won't hear from them again. This doesn't necessarily mean they don't care about you. They may simply be unable to cope with illness and the possibility of death.

Many friends fall into the category of sheer discomfort. They want to help, but they have never dealt with illness before and have no idea how to proceed. They are afraid of saying or doing the wrong thing. The last thing they want to do is make you feel worse, and often they don't realize the depth of change the cancer has caused. What most people are waiting for is your guidance. They want you to tell them what you need, whether it's a regular walk together on the beach, a weekly phone call (during which you may not want to talk about cancer), or the offer to run an occasional errand.

You will also find the odd person who disagrees vehemently with the choices you have made during treatment and recovery. Friends of this kind may have rigid ideas about diet, exercise, stress, or any number of other things.

"Some of my friends thought traditional Chinese medicine was a waste of time and money. Yet it's been incredibly helpful for me. We just don't talk about it anymore. They don't ask me about my recovery and I don't tell them."

— Tim, 28 years old, testicular cancer, 2-month survivor

Your friends want you to get well. They may, however, express this desire in less than desirable ways. Their ideals about what you require to heal may not agree with yours. Other people's judgement of your choices can be disconcerting when what you really need is reassurance. You and your friend may agree to disagree in the end, or your friend's behaviour may cause a deep rift in the relationship.

> *"Our society expects people with cancer to be so diligent now, to eat well, sleep eight to ten hours, not to drink. I felt criticized by everyone. People were telling me what to eat or that I wasn't exercising enough. I needed to find my own way. It gets on your nerves after a while."*
>
> — Karl, 46 years old, lymphoma, 6-month survivor

In each decade of our lives there are recognizable milestones, such as graduation, marriage, and starting a family. For many young adult cancer survivors, those markers get overturned. While friends go on with their lives, you may feel disconnected from them. It is common to feel angry and envious when life seems to move forward so smoothly for them and not for you.

> *"My best girlfriend just got married, another friend was having a baby, and both of my brothers bought houses. I felt left out. My life didn't seem to be progressing along the normal path, and this bothered me. It made me feel different from everyone else."*
>
> — Mary-Beth, 32 years old, leukemia, 2-year survivor

After cancer you may also feel out of sync with your friends' attitudes. While they're saying, "Come on, you've survived, it's time to enjoy life," you might not feel so carefree yet. You may be frustrated or angry, missing the old familiar connections. Your friends won't understand what you're going through unless they've been there themselves, and although it's not their fault, you may find it difficult to relate to their interests. What's important to them may no longer be so to you.

> *"I've had this life-threatening experience and what I really want to talk about is the purpose and preciousness of life, and the gratitude I feel for each day. I don't want to talk about what someone is wearing, where they're going shopping and what they're going to buy. I've just been ripped*

apart at the seams, and their worst problem is not getting the right paint
colour for their kitchen wall."

— Brittany, 39 years old, cervical cancer, 1-year survivor

It is difficult too when friends don't want to talk about cancer anymore. You may be struggling with fatigue, early menopause, or depression, but because your friends don't see any physical problems when they look at you, they want you to move on and join in other conversations. After a while, some may even stop asking you how you feel. This is when talking with others who have had cancer and share your concerns can prove invaluable.

Part of redefining normal involves finding a balance in your life. You'll want to make time for serious introspection, but sometimes it's healthier just to go to a movie. You do not have to participate in intense conversations about life all the time, either. There's nothing wrong with talking to friends about your kids, a creative project, or the books you're reading. Some days you may want to say, "This is a no-cancer day. Let's talk about something else."

The recovery process can be exhausting for everyone. You may find yourself handling each relationship differently, treading lightly around people's cancer comfort zones. You're strong for the friends who fall apart around you, silent for those who can't accept the situation, and stoic for the people who say, "Don't worry, you'll be fine."

Ultimately, cancer pushes you to take a close look at your friendships. Some survivors use this time of transition to re-examine how much they invest in certain relationships. Do you spend time with people because you have to, or because you want to? Do certain relationships give you energy and others steal it from you? Now is the time to weigh these things for yourself. You may have made some new friendships since the cancer was diagnosed. Some long-time friendships may have become deeper and more sustaining. Some relationships may be broken, though, and will not get better no matter what you do. It can be freeing to let these go.

 SELF SCAN QUESTIONS 12, 13 AND 14 *(see page 176)*

Your Relationships at Work: How's Your Day Job?

Our work is often strongly connected to our self-esteem as well as to how others perceive us. We may receive acknowledgment, recognition, respect and a sense of accomplishment from our jobs, as well as financial remuneration for our efforts. Our colleagues may also be our primary social group. For many survivors, returning to work or remaining at work is an essential step in integrating the new normal. Others begin to question their relationship to their job just as they have questioned other important relationships in their life.

We spend a lot of our lives at our jobs, and you see time from a new perspective after surviving cancer. Putting hours and hours into work that is unsatisfactory may now seem impossible. Some survivors find they need to re-evaluate the treadmill aspect of their jobs. Your side effects may cause physical limitations, cognitive changes, or emotional volatility, all of which can affect your ability to return to work or to perform your job duties adequately. Other survivors may find that, although their capabilities are intact, their priorities have changed or the stress of the job is no longer acceptable. Having cancer may give you the reason as well as the permission you need to leave an unfulfilling or undesirable job.

Sometimes it will be possible to redefine your job by using different skills or by bringing your work into better alignment with your values. Some survivors reduce or change their hours, clarify their new role in the company and adjust their responsibilities to fit their priorities. Others are motivated to reorganize their careers in order to spend more time on hobbies they love or so that they can contribute to society in other ways.

> *"I couldn't afford to quit my job, but by working three-quarters time I was able to start doing some volunteer work. My volunteer work is very satisfying and a nice complement to the work I do."*
> — Margie, 45 years old, ovarian cancer, 3-year survivor

Some survivors decide to change their attitudes, not their jobs. When you begin to see your work environment and your colleagues in a different light, you may notice subtle shifts in how you are interacting with each other.

"I was working with a couple of very difficult managers who used to really bother me. After the cancer, I thought, this really doesn't matter. I was able to let stuff go. And it's funny; it totally improved my relationship with these people."

— Annie, 51 years old, melanoma, 2-year survivor

Some cancer survivors believe it was their work that sustained their mental health and sense of normalcy throughout treatment. They love their jobs and either never stopped working or are eager to return once the treatments are over. You may be someone whose work gives you a deep sense of accomplishment, joy and self-confidence. Re-evaluating your job only reconfirms that you are working in the right situation.

Your relationships with your co-workers may also need to be re-evaluated once you're back at work. Because the workplace is an important source of social contact and personal validation, it can be surprising and hurtful if some of your colleagues now seem to ignore you or to pretend that nothing has changed. Some may simply say, "Welcome back," and never acknowledge further that your absence was due to cancer.

It is safe to assume that most of your co-workers are uncertain how to proceed. They may feel awkward, unsure of whether or not to raise the topic of your cancer. They don't want to upset you but don't know how to show their support. They may feel remaining silent is their only option at the moment.

But since cancer is so prevalent, some co-workers may also seek you out with questions about newly diagnosed family members or friends. They may feel they can talk to you about what they're going through since you've been there. It may even be their way of showing support. You may find this situation draining and upsetting, or see it as healing and empowering. Either way, it's up to you to decide whether you will choose to share your story or not.

 SELF SCAN QUESTIONS 15 AND 16 *(see page 176)*

ENDINGS AND BEGINNINGS

After an experience with cancer, society puts pressure on us to resume our former roles at work, with friends, and in the family. But cancer tends to change the rules. Survivors often discover that they have been wearing masks in the shape of what others want them to be, and it's time for the masks to come off. Others take the opportunity to reconfirm that they enjoy the roles they've assumed and the relationship choices they've made.

It takes courage to move in a new direction. Sometimes the changes you decide to make are not minor detours but a full re-routing of your life: quitting your job, moving to a new country, leaving your partner — in short, turning your life upside-down. Once you take the time to consider how cancer has touched your relationships, you can better evaluate where you want to go and who you want to take with you along this journey of recovery.

SELF SCAN NUMBER 4: ASSESSING YOUR RELATIONSHIPS

Roles and expectations

1. How do your expectations of yourself differ from other people's expectations of you?
2. Do you feel a pressure to return to the old you, the person you were before cancer? If so, from whom?
3. In what ways have the expectations of others affected your recovery?

Your relationship with yourself

4. What are the differences, big or small, between how you see or feel about yourself now and how you did before the cancer?
5. How has the cancer experience defined who you are now?

Your relationship with your partner

6. If you have a partner, how has the cancer experience changed your relationship?
7. How has having cancer affected your communication with your partner?

Your relationships with your family

8. How has the cancer experience changed your relationship with your family?
9. Are you satisfied with the way you and your family communicate, particularly in the area of concerns and expectations regarding recovery? If not, can you establish a time and place to discuss your needs and listen to the concerns of others?

Your relationships with your children

10. If you have children, how has your relationship with them changed since the cancer experience?
11. What change in actions or habits have you observed in your children since your cancer diagnosis?

Your relationships with your friends

12. How has your relationship with your friends changed since the cancer experience?

13. Which friendships have deepened? Which have become more superficial? Which have ended?

14. How have these changes affected you? What emotions come up as you think about each of these people?

Your relationships at work

15. Have you changed the way you think about your work? How so?

16. How do co-workers treat you? Do they tend to ignore you or have they genuinely engaged you in discussion about your cancer experience? How do their reactions make you feel?

CONCLUSION

It's All Connected

The Self Scans in this section of the book represent the four corners of recovery. Although cancer happens to your body, it also has a profound effect on your thoughts and emotions, your spirit, and your relationships. Answering the questions each Self Scan poses will allow you to explore these different aspects of your life as a cancer survivor.

Ultimately, healing requires you to recover the connections to all parts of yourself. The word "holistic" derives from the word "whole." While there is no single definition of holistic health, it is understood as an approach to health that treats the whole person. Researchers in the area of psycho-neuroimmunology have been learning about complex relationships among the psychological, neurological, endocrine and immune processes. To put it simply: everything is connected.

Many survivors attest to how their emotional states — their thoughts, beliefs and feelings — have a significant effect on their physical healing and vice-versa. For example, pain and fatigue can trigger emotions such as depression, anxiety, and despair, which in turn can negatively affect our relationships. The emotional and spiritual pain we experience through fear, sadness, pain, despair or a loss of faith can compound our physical suffering. Loss can trigger a negative cycle of increased fatigue, which drains our energy and sparks fear, which can cause insomnia, which increases fatigue, and so on. Conversely, our physical health improves when we feel supported by spiritual resources and loving relationships. Feeling positive about recovery and the future can lessen your fear, increase your trust in tomorrow and decrease your pain and fatigue.

The sadness, loss, and changes in roles and expectations that accompany cancer have an undeniable impact on every aspect of your life. But the interconnectedness of mind, body and spirit definitely has a bright side. Positive emotions and behaviours can lead to improved health.

Let's look at joy. What happens when you are happy? In his book *Anatomy of an Illness*, Norman Cousins reports that joyful laughter causes the brain to produce endorphins, which in turn help relieve stress and activate the immune system. (1) Activities that stimulate your senses — such as listening to music, eating something delicious or sharing a laugh with a good friend can boost your energy and lighten your spirits.

Happy people suffer as many of life's ups and downs as anyone else. The difference is that they turn to positive feelings such as appreciating the people and things they love to help them respond to setbacks. The more we practise our positive emotions, the more energy we build up to combat our fears. And combating fear leads to a reduction in things like pain and fatigue. The vicious circle can also be on our side.

Many survivors find spirituality to be an essential part of their healing process. It brings them the comfort and strength that are essential in addressing the physical and emotional challenges of cancer and its treatment. A central part of spirituality is the concept of living in the present moment. We are seldom fully present and are more likely to be thinking about our lives than living them. Conscious living is part of a deep knowing that can help mitigate the effects of illness. With conscious living you become fully aware of your body, mind, spirit and relationships with others. Once you have done the four Self Scans, you'll have taken an important step in that direction.

As we move now to talk about the process of Discovery, we will be looking at health in the broadest sense. This kind of health rebuilds your body, renews your mind and heart, restores your spirit and reaffirms your social relations. It makes space for both happiness and sadness. It teaches compassion for physical limitations and yet allows you to commit to living your life to the fullest. It is holistic, giving you the best chance of picking up all the pieces of your life and integrating them into a new, fuller picture of yourself.

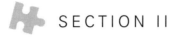 SECTION II

Framing in the Edges: Discovery

RECOVERING A SENSE OF CONTROL

CHAPTER NINE

Doorways to Change

"Without a doubt the hardest loss of all, physically and psychologically, was the loss of control. They could cut my body, my hair could fall out, but to take away my ability to be in control of my life was unbearably painful. I felt everything was slipping away, little by little, and it left a large emotional wound."

— Anne-Marie, 36 years old, breast cancer, 10-month survivor

"Mostly what I craved was connection. I really wanted to talk to people who were struggling with the same things I was, who had been there and had recovered to tell their stories. I needed a place of comfort and understanding, where there was no more pretending."

— Rebecca, 48 years old, ovarian cancer, 2-month survivor

During the process of Inquiry, you reviewed your four corners of body, mind, spirit, and relationships, using the Self Scans to establish a baseline of your current needs and concerns. Over the course of your recovery, you will be using this baseline to monitor change and track your progress.

In this second phase — Discovery — you will begin to explore the myriad choices available to you. Exploration means sorting through the confusion of such questions as *What should I do?* and *What do I want to do?* in order to make your own decisions. These explorations will help you think about healthy choices as well as encourage you to consider options that have just begun to beckon. The chapters in this section will also help you to develop new adaptive strategies.

During this phase, you will create a Healing Plan that tackles issues from your four corners and starts to frame in the edges of your recovery picture. Then you will look at the bigger picture of possibilities for your life and craft a Vision Statement for yourself. The goal of the Discovery Phase is to help you recover a sense of control and to assist you in bringing your ideas of living well closer to becoming a reality.

CONTROL: A NECESSARY ILLUSION

With the diagnosis of cancer comes an exposure to death that many survivors describe as leaving them feeling stunned or powerless. And once you enter the world of treatment, you experience a significant loss of control over your body and your life. Oncologist and president of the British Columbia Cancer Agency, Dr. Simon Sutcliffe, empathizes: "The environment of the cancer clinic is very controlling, and we do make patients extremely dependent on us, because everything is scheduled and done at our direction. After treatment ends, they are left on their own to regain control and struggle with piecing life back together." (1)

This loss of control can shake you to the core. As 46-year-old Brian, a one-year survivor of stomach cancer, describes: "It was terrifying. I had always been a pretty level-headed, controlled kind of guy, and suddenly I was experiencing fear, anxiety and helplessness." Some survivors respond to these feelings by trying to control everything they can. Others surrender to the lack of control and discover it can be a positive experience to go with the flow. Still others are able to assume control of their lives for the first time.

> *"I never felt I had control before in my life. I was just a pawn on the chess board, getting moved around by whoever was playing. Cancer made me realize I could make my own moves."*
>
> — Patricia, 30 years old, lymphoma, 2-year survivor

Through our habits and our structured routines, we build a protective shield around ourselves that gives us a sense of order. This shield helps us to feel safe, affords some degree of predictability, and allows us to proceed through life without worrying about everything that could go wrong. But after cancer you understand only too well that control is often an illusion. Even more, it is a paradox: the more you try to influence the people and events in your life, the more you discover how little control you actually have. In order to move on, however, you do need to take action to rebuild that protective shield and regain some control over your life. Taking charge is an important step in the healing process. It is a way to restore order to a life that feels chaotic.

> *"I made decisions that I could control: changing my diet, getting enough sleep, choosing my friends. I couldn't control my body and the cancer, but at least I could take charge of my environment."*
> — Hailey, 28 years old, melanoma, 18-month survivor

Regaining a sense of control can be particularly challenging if you were living a healthy life, pleased with the choices you were making, and got cancer anyway.

> *"I couldn't pinpoint what I had done to cause the cancer, so I couldn't really figure out what to add or eliminate in my lifestyle to make sure it didn't come back. What should I change? What should I not change? I was lost. How could I move forward when I was so uncertain of what to do?"*
> — Trevor, 53 years old, prostate cancer, 1-year survivor

During the Discovery Phase of your recovery, these are the kinds of questions you'll be asking yourself.

We Control with Our Choices

Crisis can either expose you to new opportunities for growth or shut you down. It is important to realize that, as a cancer survivor, you are not powerless. Although it's true that you can't control the disease, you can still learn to live well with the experience. You can even regain control over the fear that may be preventing you from moving forward.

> *"I tried to suppress the fear, but I was terrified of the cancer recurring.*
> *Finally I decided not to give it so much power. Instead I started empower-*
> *ing myself by learning how cancer works, what my chances of a recurrence*
> *were, and what lifestyle changes I could make that would increase my odds*
> *of living cancer-free. Little by little, with each positive move I made, I began*
> *to feel more in control."*
>
> — Harold, 62 years old, lung cancer, 2-year survivor

Control is the opposite of helplessness. Taking control is based on the belief that you can positively influence what happens in your life. Your readiness to act, to step up to the plate and take a swing at what life sends you, involves taking risks. It means doing whatever is necessary to own your life rather than to be a victim of circumstance.

In any situation, you can choose to be bitter or you can choose to be better. You can't choose whether or not to have cancer, but you can choose how you live with it. You can pursue what fulfills you, whether in small ways or large. Regardless of your limitations, you can find happiness and meaning in the choices you make — in how you live your life.

In his inspiring book *Man's Search for Meaning,* Dr. Viktor Frankl wrote that despite the atrocities he experienced in the Nazi concentration camps, the guards could not control his attitude: "Everything can be taken from a man but one thing; the last of human freedoms is to choose one's attitude in any given set of circumstances, to choose one's own way." (2) It is liberating to realize you have control over the lens through which you view your life. You *can* take charge of your reactions.

Opening yourself to new possibilities may require a fundamental shift in the way you think. Deep down you may feel powerless and resigned to a life of illness. You may feel you can do nothing about your health, particularly in the future. You may long to make new choices but fear the personal changes that will be required. This sense of being trapped in your life causes fear, grief and depression.

"I wasn't sure where to start. I was so afraid of the cancer and afraid of the choices I would make — what if they were wrong and the cancer did recur? My future seemed so small, and cancer such a big part of it."

— Russell, 58 years old, bladder cancer, 3-month survivor

During transition it is normal to feel disoriented. In the journey of your life you've left one way station (your pre-cancer life) but have not yet arrived at the next one. It's as if you're walking through the dark forest and can't see any path. Luckily, assuming responsibility for your own recovery program will allow you to forge your path through that forest.

You are the only one who knows which choices are right for you. To respond to your own needs you must be true to your core — the well you — and that process begins not with an act of will but with willingness. When you make choices and act upon them, you renew your trust in your own authority. When you choose to learn to live *with* the cancer, not live in fear of it, you are empowering yourself and de-powering the role cancer has in your current life. As one survivor succinctly states, "Yes, I've had cancer, but I refuse to have the focus for the rest of my life be death — it's not about dying, it's about living!"

Control What You Can

Throughout this book we will be reminding you that healing is not about fixing: it's about changing. The recovery process involves understanding what you can do for your health at various stages, whether that means gathering information, pursuing specific health care services or taking action to change unhealthy behaviour. There is no step-by-step recipe for attaining a greater sense of control. It will happen gradually and be reinforced by each new decision you make. Figuring out what you need will take time and courage. You will learn to trust your own decisions by building on your strengths and abilities, acknowledging your limitations and allowing yourself to be guided by your own needs and wants.

"No one can change it for you; no one can fix it for you. You have to make choices that fit, trust in them and then get on with your life."

— Tabitha, 51 years old, lymphoma, 25-year survivor

Living a healthy life does not guarantee you will never get sick. Survivors come to realize that certainty is an elusive concept. Eventually, most people are able to accept that life will unfold as it will. They take charge of what they can and move with the forces beyond their control.

BECOMING RESPONSE-ABLE

Each of us is responsible for our own well-being, and becoming an active participant in your own health means making conscious choices. The word *responsibility* can be divided in half — *response-ability* — to show that it involves the ability to respond. It means finding out what you need and then empowering yourself to go out and get it. Developing a take-charge attitude will put you on equal footing with the cancer and allow you to move forward in an effective and hopeful way.

> *"You can't breathe for anybody else, and they can't breathe for you. The only life you really can control is your own. I remember thinking I was being selfish when I was following my healing plan. But I realized if I didn't do these things I could die, and then what good would I be to anybody? My kids wouldn't have a mother and my husband wouldn't have a wife."*
> — Esther, 38 years old, cervical cancer, 3-year survivor

There are three key steps to becoming an active participant in your recovery process:

- Educate yourself
- Assemble your resources
- Take positive action

Educate Yourself: Knowledge Is Power

Some survivors have discovered how important it is for them to be informed. They are keen researchers and read voraciously. They want all the information they can get their hands on — even if it's downright frightening. They seek out information from medical journals, internet sources, libraries, and any other source they can find. They need the information for reassurance and to feel in control again.

> *"Afterwards, I tried to pretend it was all behind me, like it didn't happen. I ignored it and suppressed the fear, but often I was terrified of it recurring. I decided to learn how cancer works, what my chances of a recurrence were, what lifestyle factors I could do that would increase my odds of living cancer-free. Little by little, with more information and each positive move I made to stay healthy, I began to feel more in control."*
>
> — Frank, 41 years old, leukemia, 2-year survivor

Other survivors want only enough information to allow them to make wise choices. And still others do not want any information at all: they find it only adds to their fears of what might happen, and they prefer to look towards the future optimistically.

There are many sources of information available to you, including the resource section at the end of this book. Finding out what you can do for yourself is taking responsibility, whether that means attending classes, tracking down books at the library, or finding the right practitioner.

> *"I find medical information unsettling and often conflicting. The studies vary on what is and isn't a carcinogen. Some days the information raises my anxiety level; other days it reduces it. But overall I feel more in control of my fears if I have a basic understanding of what I'm dealing with."*
>
> — Clyde, 56 years old, prostate cancer, 6-month survivor

Your coping style is different from your neighbour's, your sister's or that of the survivor sitting next to you. Whatever works for you is right for you. But learning as much as you can about your cancer, its treatments and its potential long-term side effects may help you feel more in control. Most of us have a tendency to magnify our fears and assume the worst, because we don't take the time to understand exactly why we are afraid. Talk to your doctor about your concerns and keep up with the latest research on your type of cancer.

Assemble Your Resources

We will be talking in more detail about support services and other resources in the next few chapters. What's important to understand first of all is that recovery does not need to be a solo journey. You can build a health care team; you can join a support group; you can surround yourself with positive people who will help you heal. There is a myriad of support services available to cancer survivors, from pain management clinics to art therapy programs, and you should take advantage of as many of them as you need.

> *"My recovery was complicated by lymphedema and the lack of good information about what I could and couldn't do to return to an active lifestyle. The lymphedema preoccupied me for the first year. I became depressed and lost hope that I would ever be active again. Eventually I found a physiotherapist that helped me immensely and joined a support group. I wish I hadn't done it on my own for so long."*
>
> — Wanda, 48 years old, breast cancer, 3-year survivor

Every decision you make about healing should suit your lifestyle and support your commitment to health. It's important to pursue your recovery in small, manageable chunks. Many survivors have an *aha!* moment when they realize that the effects of even small changes will resonate through their lives.

> *"I went to a 'young adults with cancer' retreat in Montana for a week, and it changed my life. I met other young people my age with the same problems and I knew if they were going to be okay, I'd be okay. We spent a lot of time talking about how we felt and the changes we could make. It was so eye-opening."*
>
> — Yasmin, 18 years old, brain cancer, 1-year survivor

Take Positive Action: Your Beliefs Matter

Your beliefs about healing play a key role in how you approach the recovery process. As a survivor, you'll need to restore your faith both in your body and in your capacity to heal before you can believe that your efforts will indeed pay off. Often this faith is spurred by an act of hope — making a choice that moves you forward despite significant obstacles. It is crucial to choose activities that coincide with your beliefs — not someone else's — and with what feels right for your body and your health at the time.

With her oncologist's support, Vanessa began using complementary medicine during her treatment for lymphoma. After her chemotherapy finished, she chose to continue many of the same healing activities. During her cancer experience, she had been exposed to new attitudes and approaches, and she wanted to move towards living a more holistic and wellness-oriented life. She started to understand how the simple choices she makes daily are powerful determinants of her well-being.

> *"I still go to my acupuncturist and my naturopath. I didn't pay much attention to my health before, never had to. But now I make conscious decisions about how to live a healthy life every day. I believe what I'm doing makes a difference in how I feel day to day and that it will affect my future."*
>
> — Vanessa, 41 years old, lymphoma, 4-month survivor

It is also important not to get stuck in black-and-white thinking or in worrying too much about whether you are making the right choices. Begin with small things that you can reasonably accomplish, then either celebrate your accomplishment or choose again. Gaining faith in your choices may mean asking yourself often, *Is this a healthy choice for me right now?*

Many of us have preconceived notions about what we want from life. These ideas include familial as well as cultural definitions of success, happiness and health. For many, cancer brings chaos and impairment, disrupting a previously chosen path in life. But cancer can provide the opportunity to reassess your life or to come to terms with past disappointments and poor decisions. In her inspirational book *The Places That Scare You*, author Pema Chödrön writes, "We always have a choice. We can let the circumstances of our lives harden us and make us resentful and afraid, or we can let them soften us and make us kinder." (3)

You can make new choices, create new solutions, find promise in past failures, and turn limitations into strengths in order to recreate your life in a healthier way. Each new day offers a new start, the chance either to reaffirm the choices of yesterday or to choose differently. Finding a way to take positive action will keep you moving along your chosen path.

REFRAMING FEAR

After cancer, fear can be a constant companion. It's difficult to take charge of your life if you're always looking over your shoulder. Trying new things and making new choices will mean moving into unknown territory. This can be scary. You may want to move forward, but when you actually try it, you catch yourself scrambling back to safety.

Some survivors have experienced so many losses from cancer that they fear losing anything else. They hold on tightly to a shaky sense of control, afraid to let go. Yet it's this holding on that keeps you stuck in fear. What we resist persists. Denial is a common defense mechanism for dealing with fear, as is avoidance, through keeping very busy. Both techniques provide a short-term reprieve, but ultimately they will not help you heal. Pretending that the cobra is not really in the living room will prevent you from moving forward. Although you cannot outrun or escape fear, you can choose to face it courageously, tackling it straight on some days and turning away from it on others.

In the early days following the end of your treatment, the fear of recurrence can be át its most intense. But every day between you and the diagnosis adds hope. The passage of time reinforces the point that life without cancer does exist. It is also important to realize that a recurrence does not mean certain death. Many people who have been dealt a recurrence are alive and well today.

Action Is the Antidote
The best way to push past fear is to take action. Whatever you do will make a difference. For many survivors, addressing their fears is an important starting point. Once the resistance to fear lessens, life flows more easily. Over time, most survivors find ways to reframe their fears, to accept them rather

than experiencing them as limits. When you are able to clearly identify your fear and accept it for what it is, it's like a heavy curtain going up.

"I deal with my fears of recurrence as if they were a trip to the dentist — with dread, but also with a knowledge that they will pass."
— Kate, 34 years old, ovarian cancer, 3-year survivor

As we discussed in Chapter Six, where you completed the emotional Self Scan, there are some predictable triggers of fear such as follow-up appointments and anniversary dates. Knowing what triggers your fears helps you to manage them. You may find yourself anxious in the weeks or days before your next check-up. Your friends or family members may comment that you seem unfocused or uptight. When you can name the reason behind the feeling, you begin to tame your anxiety. Plan ahead and take proactive measures for managing difficult occurrences.

"Because my follow-up visits always generate a huge mixture of emotions for me, I decided to stop trying to suppress or deny the fear and instead find ways to celebrate myself on that day. I always planned a little treat for myself after I left the hospital, whether it was getting a massage, buying a new blouse, or eating expensive chocolates."'
— Alexandra, 42 years old, thyroid cancer, 3-year survivor

Tools for Facing the Fear

Many survivors find themselves searching for something that will ground them, tools that will steady their beating hearts amidst the fear. The following tools can be used to re-establish emotional equilibrium. Some distract you from fear by shifting the focus to other activities. Others help you face the fear head on. You can use one or all of the following tools as you need to. The more coping skills you have, the more resilient you'll be.

Don't do it alone. Spending time with family and friends can help you reduce stress. Let them know that you're afraid and you need them to listen. If you're not comfortable talking with someone so close to you, reach out to other survivors. They will understand exactly what you're feeling, and you can learn a lot by hearing how others manage their fears. If fear and anxiety persist and are interfering with your daily life, seek help from a health care professional. Psychological counselling can assist you in sorting through your fears and figuring out how to deal with them.

Return to the present moment. Fear of recurrence relates to something that might happen in the future, not to something that is happening right now. Bring your awareness back to the present moment and know you are all right here and now.

Use relaxation techniques. Visualization, meditation, and breathing exercises can help you calm your anxiety, regain a sense of connection to your body and ease an overactive mind. Simply observing your breath can help you stay centred in your body when your mind is restless. And learning to breathe properly is one of the most important things you can do when you feel as if fear is taking over. Breathe in through your nose for four counts, hold for four counts and exhale for eight. You can also find a peaceful image to focus on in times of turmoil: a tranquil place in nature, a person who grounds you, or a particular object you find soothing.

You may want to take a class in order to learn meditation or visualization techniques. Some groups are aimed specifically at cancer survivors. There are also numerous relaxation tapes and CDs available in bookstores and libraries. You can listen to these during the day or in the middle of the night when the fear wells up — anytime you need to tune out the world and tune in to a restful state of being.

Be creative. When you immerse yourself in art, music, or writing, you appreciate what's before you. Your mind is caught up in the wonder and beauty of the moment. It's hard to sing and worry at the same time!

Movement. Do something physical. When you get scared, get moving. Physical activity is good for the body, but it also calms the mind. That's one of the benefits of the daily attentive walk we recommend: it gets you in motion, which requires concentration and shuts your mind off for a while. Gentle exercise like Tai Chi or yoga will also centre your breathing and ease the fear.

Keep the faith. Draw on your spiritual or religious beliefs and traditions for strength. Explore ways to focus on the larger context of life and growth and trust in the journey you are on. This may mean more frequent trips to your place of worship or engaging in regular prayer throughout the day. "I surrender" is a phrase that symbolizes giving your fear over to God's grace, knowing you'll be supported along the way.

Examine the fear closely. Learn what you are really afraid of instead of allowing vague, overwhelming worries to take over. Do you fear the physical dying process, or death itself? Some survivors work with professionals to understand the physiological changes the body goes through in the dying process. That way, they know what dying looks like, and some people find the facts reassuring. Coming to accept that death is a part of life and that no one gets out alive can help you put the cycle of life and death into perspective. Attending a workshop or retreat aimed at exploring death and dying can help you come to an understanding that fits with your beliefs.

Let go. Write a letter to the cancer and then burn it, so that the disease will no longer hold power over you. Build a clay sculpture of the cancer and then smash it, or paint the cancer in dark colours on a canvas, then paint over it with hopeful, healing colours.

Have a touchstone. Carry something with you that you can physically touch to keep you grounded. Place a smooth rock you collected off the beach in your pocket, carry a fuzzy good luck charm in your purse, leave rosary beads next to your bed, play with a special charm on your bracelet, or wear beautiful Tibetan worry beads.

Use a mantra or affirmation. If you repeat the same negative phrase over and over in your head, your fear can escalate out of control. The idea of a mantra, which can be one word or a full phrase, is to interrupt the negative cycle of fear and worry and replace it with something that's calming. When your mind starts obsessing, stop it with a mantra. Here are a few examples survivors use:

- Stop
- Very slowly
- Thy will be done
- Keep moving
- Hold it together
- This too shall pass
- The Hail Mary prayer
- The Serenity Prayer — God grant me the serenity to accept the things I cannot change, the courage to change the things I can, and the wisdom to know the difference.

FROM RECOVERY TO WELLNESS

While there is an abundance of information available about health and well-ness, it is ultimately up to you to decide what will meet your current health care needs and give you the greatest benefit. Certainly what is helpful to one person — group support, meditation, or herbal remedies — may not work for another. To create a personalized Healing Plan, you may need to explore activities you've never tried before. Consider this a period of experimenta-tion. Challenging your old habits is part of finding the answers, motivation, and support you need.

"Wellness" is an ancient, multidimensional concept that views health as a dynamic, ever-changing process. Such an attitude focuses on what's right with us rather than what's wrong. It is based on the belief that the interaction of our mind, body and spirit — what we think, do, value, and believe in — influences our health. Wellness involves good nutrition, exercise, stress man-agement, creativity, spiritual connections, and positive social relationships.

Now is the time to reassess what contributes to your health and what takes away from it. What will create the right combination of conditions for your healing? Maybe you need to drink more water, take a dance class or volunteer at the local food bank. You will be developing a formal Healing Plan as you work through the next chapter of the book, but you can start by thinking about these questions.

In the pursuit of wellness, if you can change one unhealthy habit, you are taking a significant step forward. Alcoholics Anonymous, Weight Watchers and other behavioural change programs teach that you are more likely to succeed if you modify just one behaviour and make that change stick before moving on to the next. Remember, it takes three weeks of steady commitment and action to establish any new habit. Be patient, and allow yourself time to adjust before making additional changes.

INTENTION

As important as it is to figure out what you want to do and how you will do it, you must also ask yourself why you want to accomplish something. Every choice or decision you make is born of an intention. Your intention is the purpose you have in mind, the invisible guiding force behind your actions.

Intentions are powerful forces in our lives. They can give us the strength to overcome obstacles. However, unlike behaviour that is public and observable, our intentions are private. They remain hidden until we act.

Whether you are considering small or large choices as you recover from cancer, it is important to clarify your intentions at each step. Ask yourself *What do I honestly want from this situation?* before you act. It is equally wise to pay attention to the results of your actions. Remember, intending an action is not the same as performing one. As the old maxim goes, "The road to Hell is paved with good intentions." You may intend to go to the gym, but if you don't actually go, your intentions do not produce any results.

THE MOTIVATION CONTINUUM

Motivation after cancer tends to be based on two forces: fear and purpose. A key question to ask yourself is *Am I making choices based on health and living well, or am I trying to keep the cancer at bay?*

Fear-Based Choices ············· **Purpose-Based Choices**

Motivation is our prompt or incentive to act on chosen goals. Both ends of the continuum shown above play useful roles in motivating us to action. It is appropriate to make choices anywhere along this line, depending upon the situations in which we find ourselves. We move back and forth on the continuum our entire lives as our intentions and motivations change.

Time is also an important variable. Your intention to keep your cancer at bay may initially drive your pursuit of recovery. Fear of recurrence is a powerful motivator, and it can be a positive force.

> *"If I get a whisper from somewhere that triggers my fear, I regard it as a positive stimulus to do the work I have to do in order to stay on track."*
> — Heather, 55 years old, breast cancer, 1-year survivor

But although fear can jumpstart you into action, fears do recede over time. Eventually denial or old habits come back, and motivation decreases. Even the threat of death does not keep people committed to making changes over the long term. Furthermore, fear can easily turn into a negative force. It can immobilize you by feeding you the thought that, since you're susceptible to a recurrence, there's no point in trying to heal. It can cause panic or trigger negative emotions such as guilt and blame. If you find yourself making choices simply to stop your anxiety, it's time to take a deep breath and clarify your thinking.

If your intention around a decision is purpose-based — that is, you begin an exercise program in order to feel better, to cope with stress, and to improve your well-being — then you are likely to keep your commitment to wellness long after your fear of recurrence subsides. Think about your current activities and ask yourself what is motivating your choices. Whenever you are able to focus on wellness instead of on the disease, you are moving past fear and towards a more purpose-driven source of motivation.

"I've started going to the gym three times a week, eating well, and I've joined a writing group because I want to enjoy my life and live it in a healthy way. I'm not doing this to kill the cancer. This isn't about winning and losing; it's about living well in the time I have left."

— Aeden, 43 years old, melanoma, 2-year survivor

ENERGY BUILDERS AND DRAINERS

Moving through change is a dynamic process of learning from experience. It requires us to pay attention to both what aids and what hinders our healing. Certain aspects of our lives build our energy and bring us joy, which in turn enhances our ability to heal. Other aspects deplete our energy and cause stress, lessening our enjoyment of life and our ability to move forward.

One survivor may replenish her energy through yoga and meditation; another will find being with family and friends a source of renewal.

"Walks along the beach, or a good night's sleep, build it. Fear and worry drain it. Feeling hopeful builds it. Blaming drains it. I've finally started realizing where my energy goes and what it does to me. I notice when I leave a situation if am I exhausted or energized."

— Cindy, 33 years old, lymphoma, 6-month survivor

While you are picking up the pieces of your life, you will often be dealing with other people's issues. Be aware: your family and friends can hold great sway over you, influencing your choices and healing patterns. Unwanted advice can be a big energy drainer. Learning to say, "No, thanks, that doesn't work for me" is an empowering step forward.

Both family and friends advised Elspeth not to work so hard just after her treatment. But Elspeth loves her work and finds great healing in it. For her, work is not the stressor others assume it to be.

"People have their own ideas about what's good for you. My mother-in-law urged me to take up meditation, but I want to try creative cooking. I found if you don't do what others say, you feel guilty, as if you're letting

*them down. It becomes another burden. I'm learning to stand tall and not
let myself be forced into following everyone's 'helpful' suggestions."*
— Elspeth, 54 years old, breast cancer, 2-month survivor

You know best what ignites your healing spirit. Before embarking on the creation of your Healing Plan, you may find it helpful to make a list in your recovery journal of the things that boost and drain your energy, physically and emotionally.

My Energy Drainers	*My Energy Builders*
1.	1.
2.	2.
3.	3.
4.	4.

Include both activities and people. What impact do your current relationships have on your energy? Do you turn to spirituality to recharge your batteries? Or does an evening with friends accomplish that? Some people find that solitude and a good book energize them. For others it's creating a sumptuous meal for twelve. If you never renew your energy, you will eventually have nothing left to give. Knowing what builds you up is essential to your health and peace of mind.

*"Sometimes energy builders and drainers are the same people. My best
friend, who has been a big support for me throughout my treatments,
doesn't share my new 'seize the day' attitude. I've found I spend more time
with friends who bring out the new spontaneous side of me."*
— Carla, 31 years old, leukemia, 1-year survivor

MAKE CHANGES FOR YOURSELF

Throughout this healing journey, it is important to be as true to yourself as possible. You are the one who had cancer. You are the one who needs to heal. Each of us does things at our own pace. Some survivors need to make quick decisions, whereas others are cautious and prefer to take their time.

In the next chapter we will look at four approaches to healing that can assist you in making concrete plans for regaining your health. Your Healing Plan will address your various side effects. Then we will throw open the door to possibility and see what you can envision for your life after cancer.

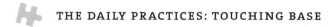

Attentive Walking

Some days, no matter your route, your walk may seem all uphill. Take a minute to notice how you inhale and exhale, whether you take full, deep breaths or quick, shallow ones. As you inhale, try to let your chest expand and your ribs rise; feel your chest relax and your shoulders lower as you exhale. Breathe in all that is good in the world and breathe out the pain and sadness. Lengthen your exhalations to let go of tension, and then rest with the quiet feeling of being in the moment. Now bring your awareness gently back to your surroundings. *Just keep walking.*

The Five-Question Check-In

As you answer your five-question check-in, notice which questions test your willingness to record the raw truth. Remember, your answers are for your eyes only. You can be as rude, as honest, as fearful, or as courageous as you want to be when you write in your recovery journal. Writing is a terrific form of therapy. Don't be afraid to use it.

CHAPTER TEN

Four Approaches to Healing: Designing a Healing Plan

"What I love about the music and dance is that it takes me totally away from my mind. It is not something you do with your intellect. You must put your whole self into it."

— Alma, 43 years old, ovarian cancer, 9-month survivor

"I joined a group of men, all cancer survivors, who were canoeing down some of the worlds' largest rivers. Our intent is to spread the word that there is life after cancer — a good life — and to demonstrate that survivors are active, strong and hopeful."

— Joseph, 29 years old, testicular cancer, 2-year survivor

The next piece in the recovery puzzle involves designing a Healing Plan that will build on your strengths and address your limitations as well as attending to what boosts or drains your energy. Your Healing Plan will set out your intentions and chart a course of action for healing during your recovery.

Through the Inquiry process you learned to listen to your body, to feel rather than resist the day-to-day fluctuations of energy, symptoms, and emotions that accompany the healing process. Healing occurs on many levels. It includes heeding your intuition, supporting positive choices, and making decisions that respect your changing state of health.

Your Healing Plan is intended to address your side effects, but remember that these are not just physical. Mood swings, marital problems, and spiritual angst can all appear as a result of cancer. If you are still adjusting to the side effects of treatment, your Healing Plan will likely centre initially on physical concerns; you might concentrate on managing your fatigue or walking pain-free for a few blocks. If you are a survivor further along in your recovery, you may choose to focus primarily on emotional, spiritual or relationship concerns. Since every survivor's needs are different, this chapter presents four different approaches to healing. We suggest that, as you read about these, you make some notes in your recovery journal about what might work for you. At the end of the chapter, you'll have a chance to put your own Healing Plan down on paper, using one of these four approaches or a combination.

Because dealing with side effects can sometimes evoke anger, frustration and blame, we'll be encouraging you to include safe avenues for self-expression in your Healing Plan. Dancing, gardening, exercise, counselling, and wedging clay are all examples of healthy outlets. They will help you move from using defensive mechanisms such as denial, withdrawal and passivity to a place of strength where you can say *I may not like this, but I can handle it.*

> *"I felt as if life were a movie and I was just standing still and watching as others moved on — getting married, having kids, getting great jobs. Defining my healing goals gave me a lead part — the role of main character — in my life."*
> — Darla, 26 years old, melanoma, 7-month survivor

Having a Healing Plan can help you stay focused during difficult times. Working with a plan will build your resilience so that you can address the multiple fears and "dark nights of the soul" that continue long after the treatments are over. Remember: simple actions can be powerful healing vehicles, and they are often easier to commit to than elaborate plans. Finding frequent opportunities for ten minutes of good belly laughing may give you more comfort than following a complicated diet. Sitting with your cat, walking the dog or drawing with your child may all be perfect antidotes to stress-filled mornings. Only you know what you truly need.

THE ART OF HEALING

Thank goodness for the scientific researchers of this world who explore the ways survivors are diagnosed, treated, and monitored. They establish clinical treatment guidelines, identify and control the acute and late effects of cancer, and establish successful recovery monitoring tools. But much of the art of healing occurs outside the field of science. It encompasses all of who you are.

Healing from within by connecting to every aspect of yourself is the key to a successful recovery program. Just as a work of art expresses an artist's full creative powers, so will your recovery call on your full inner resources. The art lies in how you choose to express yourself in the process.

CREATING YOUR OWN HEALTH CARE TEAM

Before we move to looking at the four approaches to healing, we want to mention a key component of any Healing Plan: your personal health care team. While it is important to trust your doctor, you must become a partner in your own care, advocating on your own behalf to get the information, expertise, and care or service you need. In order to alleviate anxiety and stay well, it is important to advise your doctor of aches and pains, emotional volatility, or other significant changes to your health and well-being. However, often a family physician won't have the time or expertise to answer all of your physical, emotional and spiritual concerns. In fact, it is unreasonable to expect one individual to be able to address such a myriad of issues. What you need is a community of experts to support you as your life changes. This is your health care team.

As more and more survivors design their own recovery programs, it is becoming common for them to build their own recovery teams. Your team can provide you with information, compassion, and various resources as they work with you to address your unique recovery needs. As you develop good communication with these various individuals and share in the decision-making process, you begin to recover a sense of control over your health.

Your team can be as small as you and your doctor, but it will usually expand to include people such as other health practitioners, a spiritual advisor, or a personal trainer. Consider the benefits to your recovery of consulting a nutritionist, a yoga instructor, an acupuncturist, a naturopath, a massage therapist, a physiotherapist, an occupational therapist, a counsellor or psychiatrist, a member of the clergy, or a life coach.

When you build your own health care team, you are taking charge of your current recovery as well as committing to a healthy future. Samira manages her side effects with a team comprised of her family doctor, a nutritionist, an acupuncturist, and a rabbi. Her team changed with her needs.

"Initially, I had a counsellor on my team. Although I only went for eight sessions, the counselling was excellent. It helped me change a lot of my attitudes that had been really getting in my way."

— Samira, 34 years old, lymphoma, 5-month survivor

Be assertive in your relationship with your health care team. If someone is not meeting your needs, find another person who does. Your team should be composed of people who are empowering and fully on your side, people who express both hope and optimism. Every member of your team should inspire confidence in you and support your choices to heal. Remember: the most important person on your health care team is YOU.

THE FOUR APPROACHES TO HEALING

In our research we have discovered four general approaches to healing: the Physical Approach, the Connected Approach, the Creative Approach and the Contributing Approach. Many of the survivors we've interviewed use one or more of these — often refining them through trial and error — to navigate through the post-treatment Void and regain a sense of control in their lives. We've included their experiences and suggestions here to stimulate your own ideas.

As you read through the four approaches, pay attention to the ideas that appeal to you. Keep in mind that some survivors choose to concentrate on one healing approach, while others create plans that combine elements from two, three or all four. Enjoy the freedom of discovery. You may be surprised to discover what you would actually *like* to do in the name of ongoing healing. Be curious and open, but recognize this is an important exploration: you might just find a missing piece that fits into your wellness puzzle. Now is also a good time to look at the baseline you created during the Inquiry process. An important clue might lie in which Self Scan you chose to do first.

Again, we recommend that you write down any ideas or suggestions you might want to pursue in your recovery journal. These will form the basis of your own Healing Plan.

1. THE PHYSICAL APPROACH

Dealing with the physical side effects from cancer and its treatment is the first priority for many survivors. You may be looking for a way to manage fatigue, pain, or sleep disturbances in order to resume your routines as quickly as possible. Gathering information about your condition and then working closely with your health care team is essential in the physical approach to healing.

Managing Side Effects

It is hard to move forward when you are experiencing debilitating physical side effects. The good news is that most side effects can be effectively managed. The first step you can take is to appreciate the full impact of your side effects on your life, overriding the natural tendency to avoid, ignore or downplay them.

One of the purposes of the Self Scans you completed during the Inquiry process was to help you clarify your current and potential side effects. The more you know about what causes and relieves them and about how to prevent further complications, the better able you will be to address them. There are numerous books, pamphlets and online resources available on specific side effects. We've listed some that we feel are useful in our resource section.

Addressing Aches and Pains

A fear of recurrence can cause each ache and pain to send shivers down your back. For most concerns, remember the two-week rule: if your symptoms persist for two weeks or more, consult your physician and get them checked out. Most often these symptoms are due to something else, but taking a proactive approach in monitoring your aches and pains is always wise. Constantly looking for changes which might indicate that the cancer has recurred can drive you crazy and cause obsessive behaviour, but ignoring substantial changes — the ostrich effect — isn't a smart approach to your health at any stage of life. As time moves on, you will feel less worried about life's daily bumps and bruises and gain a new perspective on managing your care.

The Complements

Research has shown that more than half of all cancer survivors use complementary approaches to reduce stress, manage side effects, and prevent a cancer recurrence. Complementary therapies are concerned primarily with stimulating the body's natural ability to heal itself. Some focus on the mind-body connection through such activities as biofeedback, breathing exercises, visualization, meditation, guided imagery, progressive muscle relaxation, hypnosis, journalling, yoga, Tai chi, and Qigong. Others combine a physical intervention with energy work, diet, exercise, and vitamins. The full range of complementary approaches is too diverse to list here, but some of the most common include homeopathy, acupuncture, naturopathy, therapeutic touch, osteopathy, aromatherapy, traditional Chinese medicine, and macrobiotics.

Many survivors feel that by investigating approaches outside of conventional medicine, they regain control of their own health; that in turn gives them hope. It can be empowering to research, choose and use the therapies that appeal to you. By expanding the possible healing options, complementary therapies broaden our horizons and ultimately enhance our quality of life.

Taking Charge of Your Physical Health

Diet and exercise are two areas of life that are within our control. Research shows that good nutrition and regular exercise make a significant difference in how we feel and how we react to stress. Maintaining a healthy body weight through diet and exercise helps reduce the risk of developing many diseases including some cancers. Good nutrition and regular exercise can improve well-being and help cancer survivors cope with common side effects such as fatigue and weight gain.

You Are What You Eat

Our relationship with food is a complicated one for most of us, and that is even more true after cancer. Your diet provides nutrients that promote healing, repair damaged tissues and clear toxic substances from your system. Yet survivors are so inundated with conflicting information about diet that the majority complain of being confused about what to eat or what not to eat in order to heal from cancer and prevent a recurrence.

Re-establishing the delight of eating after cancer treatment is very important. Our food is meant to be savoured while at the same time providing nourishment and sustenance. Following a balanced, practical and delicious diet gives you a greater likelihood of success.

Studies show that people with diets rich in fruits and vegetables and low in fat have a lower incidence of cancer. If you have not followed a healthy diet in the past, this is a perfect opportunity for you to initiate a few changes. Start small: switch from whole milk to skim, eat one more fruit or vegetable every day, or substitute yogurt for mayonnaise. Experiment with substitutes in your favourite recipes, such as using olive oil instead of butter or whole grain rice instead of white. Change doesn't have to be earth-shattering in order to be effective. In fact, you are far more likely to stick with small changes than large ones.

Many survivors decide to stock their kitchens with an assortment of healthy staples. Some consult a nutritionist to learn more about food and its role in sustaining health. Some people plant herb gardens so they will have access to fresh herbs all year round. You can take cooking classes, explore culinary websites or buy new cookbooks to inspire you to eat healthily.

The basic principles of all healthy eating plans include:

- eating five or more servings of fruits and vegetables every day
- limiting sweets and salt intake

- eating more high-fibre foods
- reducing saturated fats
- limiting alcohol consumption
- eating a variety of foods
- limiting your consumption of red meats, especially high-fat or processed meats
- eating fewer smoked, salted, and nitrate-cured foods

Above all, enjoy your food choices.

> *"The further I get away from cancer, the less broccoli I eat. Today I try to eat well, but I'm not wildly obsessed about it the way I used to be. I actually came to the conclusion after two years of no booze, no chocolate, no coffee, no nothing, that part of what I enjoy about life is coffee. So why not have a coffee once in a while?"*
> — Archie, 52 years old, bladder cancer, 2-year survivor

Move Your Body

Many survivors are uncertain about how to mend their bodies after treatment. *How much exercise is too much? How much is too little? Can I damage anything if I begin too soon or work out too hard? Will I set myself back if I don't start exercising?* These are all valid questions.

Medical exercise guidelines are constantly being challenged. Gone are the days when doctors advised patients to rest for long periods of time or to refrain from returning to activities they love. Today, survivors begin range-of-motion programs almost immediately after surgery and participate in gradual strength-training programs and gentle aerobic exercise even during chemotherapy or radiation.

More and more, research is concluding that exercise is a good way to prevent a recurrence of many types of cancer. Regular exercise can elevate the body's immune system, a key factor in healing. It has even been shown to slow the growth rate of tumour cells. Many survivors use exercise as a safe way of releasing anger and of working through the fear and sadness that surface from time and time.

Movement also renews your confidence by reconnecting you with your physical self, a critical aspect of the healing process. As little as 30 minutes of low to moderately intense physical activity such as walking, cycling, or swimming most days of the week can:

- reduce symptoms of fatigue and pain
- improve your mood
- decrease anxiety and depression
- help you maintain healthy weight
- improve your cardiovascular health
- boost your self-esteem
- increase your energy levels
- improve your sleep

Fitness is a mixture of several components, including strength, endurance, flexibility, balance, and coordination. Choosing the right type of activity is important: that is, it must be right for you. The stretching and breath work that yoga affords is very healing for some people but too slow for others. The non-weight-bearing aspect of swimming makes it a good choice for those with joint problems, and ballroom or salsa dancing combines movement with socializing and can be a nice way for you to spend time with your partner. Some survivors gravitate towards gentle exercise that not only strengthens the body but calms the mind, such as Tai Chi and Qigong. Others choose more vigorous aerobic and strength-based programs such as cycling, gym classes, dance, weight-training programs and Pilates. The key to whatever you choose is to become reacquainted with your body by finding joy in movement. If you choose an activity that suits your personality, you are far more likely to stick with it.

Talk to your doctor about beginning an exercise program and then seek supervision from a trained physiotherapist, kinesiologist, personal trainer, health educator, or cancer exercise specialist, all of whom can provide you with information and expertise to help you develop a program tailored to your health and recovery goals.

Leisure Activities

Leisure activities can be an important source of joy and relaxation, but survivors find that it is not always easy to return to them right away. Sometimes this is because of medical advice. For example, breast cancer survivors used to be told to give up activities such as canoeing, tennis, and cycling, for fear that these would predispose them to lymphedema (a swelling of the arm). But researchers have found that bilateral upper body exercise, such as dragon boating and gentle, flatland cross-country skiing, can prevent and even treat lymphedema if you start slowly and work in conjunction with a defined weight-lifting program.

Most people are able to return to their former activities if they resume them slowly, gradually building up strength and endurance. You might have to take some preventive measures, such as wearing a compression sleeve or watching for signs and symptoms of complications. Consult your physician if you are unsure of whether or not it is safe to resume your former hobbies.

If you do not have a hobby you enjoy, why not consider taking up something new? Community centres abound with interesting and unusual courses that provide good introductions to a new interest. Participating with others in a shared interest is also a great way to meet people. There are now many groups composed solely of cancer survivors who fly-fish, climb mountains, race dragon boats and go hiking together. Not only will these activities help you stay in shape, they serve as powerful support groups full of information and understanding.

Hobbies can be healing. Whether you choose to take up quilting, knitting, playing the guitar, bird watching, or collecting stamps, you can find an activity that calms the mind and lifts the spirits.

Stress Management

Developing skills and ability to deal with stress and emotional turmoil is essential to building confidence in yourself and your choices. Coping with side effects in addition to the realities of everyday life leads many survivors to explore techniques for reducing stress. You might consider breathing exercises, cognitive restructuring programs, relaxation techniques, biofeedback, journal writing, meditation, gardening, music, dance, prayer or visualization.

A crucial coping strategy is to keep yourself in good physical health by eating well, getting enough rest, and setting reasonable goals about what you will accomplish each day. While it is important to stay active, remember to listen to your body and take time for yourself when you need to.

A Healing Environment

Many survivors find they need a sanctuary — a place where they can relax and replenish their depleted resources. For some people this is their home; for others it means spending more time in nature, in church, or at the family cottage. We all have different requirements for a sanctuary, but we can no doubt agree that it is difficult to heal in a place that is cluttered, loud, and busy.

> *"I realized I hadn't spent much time making my house a home, so I bought some flowers, soothing music, and fragrant candles for my living room. Then I moved the unpacked boxes downstairs into storage and cleaned up the house. Now I feel like I can settle in for a while and rest."*
> — Annette, 42 years old, lymphoma, 2-month survivor

Many survivors speak of craving physical comfort, such as a big soft chair, the right pillow, a cozy blanket, a hot bath, or a cup of hot tea. You can incorporate anything into your home environment that you think will aid your healing process: colour and fragrance, music, natural or soft lighting, and inspirational objects such as books, paintings and affirmations.

Some survivors create a special corner in a room. Others find a porch swing or a hammock to which they can retreat. Some even build studios just for meditation, relaxation, art work or journalling. In his book *Power of Myth*, Joseph Campbell encourages us: "You must have a room or a certain hour of the day where you do not know what was in the morning paper ... a place where you can simply experience and bring forth what you are, and what you might be ... At first you may find nothing happening ... But if you have a sacred place and use it, take advantage of it, something will happen!" (1)

2. THE CONNECTED APPROACH

For some survivors, the primary path to healing involves exploring their relationships with themselves, others, and/or the divine. The connected approach deals chiefly with the spiritual and social side effects of cancer.

We are each part of a vast web of interconnecting relationships: acquaintances, colleagues, family, and friends. We touch the lives of others and their lives touch ours, often in subtle ways. Many survivors feel gratitude for the support they received throughout their treatments, and some come to realize they need more support in their daily lives, be it from friends, family or other survivors who share their experiences. For them, the connected approach is ideal.

Connect with Yourself

Before you deepen your connections with others, it is important to establish a connection with yourself. Many survivors have spent a great deal of time and energy taking care of others and very little time taking care of themselves. Now is the time to take your own needs seriously. You will want to develop the ability to acknowledge your limits, as well as your strengths and potential, and to listen to the small voice within when it whispers your true healing needs and longings.

Your ultimate goal in connecting with yourself is to live from a sense of purpose rather than allowing fear to motivate your choices. This will require some solitary time that you spend either in reflection or in activities such as walking in nature, writing in your journal, painting, or gardening. Choose an activity that you love and that gives you confidence and a sense of well-being. Finding this quiet time might require a change of place. Some survivors choose to go on a spiritual retreat, to camp alone for a few days, or to escape to a friend's home when the friend is away.

The idea is to reconnect with what fills you up, be it nature, art, dance, or sewing. Find the way that is right for you, and you will ignite your healing spirit.

Reconnecting with Others

Research shows that support from family and friends has a powerful salutary effect on your emotional well-being and physical health. The better your relationships are, the better your health tends to be. Friends and family can lead by example and encourage healthier lifestyles, like following a better diet, exercising, and quitting smoking. As well, when those close to you are there in troubled times, you feel valued, loved and respected, all of which lead to decreased stress. Spending time with people you care about has been associated with improved immune function, too. Loved ones aren't just the people who call you on your birthday — they're good for you!

Some survivors find that having cancer strengthens and enhances their relationships. Others discover that they have not put the time and energy they might have into an important relationship. They decide to spend less time at work and more time with their spouse, children, parents, or friends. Perhaps you will decide that your own priorities should change. You could start taking the children to school instead of rushing to work early, or take more time off to go on holiday, or find a hobby or activity you can pursue with your loved ones.

Some survivors find it important to address unfinished business. You might decide to call an old high school friend, mend fences with your brother, or make peace with an uncle. Addressing unfinished business may mean healing old wounds or acknowledging regrets. Regrets in particular — the "if only" issues — can siphon off the energy you need for enjoying the present. But handling these issues is easier said than done. Some survivors realize they must come to terms with unpleasant events, painful disappointments, or the consequences of their own past choices — the so-called bad decisions.

Letting go of resentment will likely bring you face to face with forgiveness. Sometimes what you need is to forgive yourself, to stop blaming yourself for past indiscretions or lost opportunities. Sometimes you need to forgive others who have harmed you through ignorance, neglect, or abuse. We release ourselves and others when we let go of our grievances, judgements, and anger.

Finding forgiveness in any form is crucial for healing. To forgive is to put a period at the end of the sentence. We can't alter our past, but we can free ourselves from any oppressive shadow the past may cast by shining the light of forgiveness upon it. That is a way to live more fully in the present.

Support Groups

Even those with a close personal support network can find at times that it's not enough. Many survivors feel that friends and family can never truly understand their cancer experience. Sometimes what you need is to move beyond your immediate circle for support. You need to find a support group.

> *"I didn't want to talk about the cancer anymore with my friends and family; they've heard it all and they've moved past it. But I still needed to talk about it, so I joined an art therapy program for breast cancer survivors, and it proved to be just what I needed at this time in my recovery."*
> — Katie, 43 years old, colorectal cancer, 10-month survivor

Support groups can meet a number of needs. While men tend to use the group as a primary source of information, women often see it as an opportunity for authentic connection. In fact, such groups function on both levels. A support group offers a safe environment in which to express your fears and hopes and to be understood by others in similar situations. Survivors feel less alone and gain a sense of belonging, often for the first time since leaving the hospital. Many say their support group offered them their first opportunity to address their fears of dying, since they didn't want to scare their families with such thoughts.

A support group also functions as a forum for the latest information concerning your type of cancer. Often a health care professional is invited to speak about new research in treatment and recovery. Besides that, other survivors can be a gold mine of ideas when it comes to healing and coping skills. It has been well documented that attending a support group improves your quality of life by lessening feelings of isolation. By watching and listening to others, you might even be inspired to live a healthier life.

> *"Joining a support group at my local hospital was like buying private insurance. I felt if I could keep myself informed and stay on top of what was new, then I'd be okay. I found the group not only informational but inspiring. These people changed my life."*
> — Samantha, 46 years old, breast cancer, 1-year survivor

Support groups come in many forms, from traditional group programs to week-long workshops and weekend retreats. Cancer outreach programs can connect you by phone with another survivor whose cancer is similar to yours. This is particularly valuable for those who suffer from rare forms of cancer; it's easier to see the light at the end of your tunnel with the help of someone who's already come through.

Internet-based support groups are ideal for people who prefer to communicate online rather than face to face. In the comfort of your home, and at your convenience, you can share your story via e-mail or in a chat room and connect with others going through the same experience. Online chat groups might include newsgroups that act as virtual bulletin boards with messages to read, topics to browse and electronic mailing lists you can join. Internet-based groups are also well-suited to those who live in rural areas where access to regular support groups is difficult, or to people whose side effects or other conditions render them immobile. Other types of online support include art therapy and writing programs. In addition, there are support groups for friends and family members of survivors to help them come to grips with change, be it social, financial or physical.

Some support groups are run by professional facilitators such as counsellors, nurses, social workers, or psychologists. Other, led by group members, are known as peer or self-help groups. Some groups are run in hospitals or cancer centres, and some in the community. You can join most support groups at any time. While some specify men or women only, or are disease- or age-specific, there are also groups that accept anyone, with any type of cancer. Some groups are highly structured; others are less formal and may have a social component. Rest assured: somewhere there is a group that will meet your needs.

You can find out about the support groups in your area by contacting your hospital's social work or counselling department; asking your doctor; contacting your local community centre, library or place of worship; asking other survivors; reading the newsletters available in cancer treatment centres or cancer libraries; or calling the local office of the Canadian Cancer Society.

Professional Support

Support groups are a tremendous resource, but they might not suit your personality. Not everyone is comfortable working in a group. Many choose one-on-one support from a professional counsellor, psychologist or psychiatrist. Survivors turn to counselling to help them with problems such as depression, mood swings, unresolved issues from the past, and other emotional issues.

> *"My counsellor gave me compassion without the 'poor-you' attitude. She was just what I needed. She talked to me about reconnecting with myself, about what I wanted to do with the rest of my life, and she got me thinking about my physical and emotional needs."*
>
> — Loretta, 35 years old, leukemia, 3-year survivor

Professional guidance eases the difficult decisions you may be wrestling with during recovery. Seek a professional if you are feeling overwhelmed, are unable to concentrate, are not eating or sleeping, are not communicating with your friends or family, are feeling isolated, or just need someone to jumpstart your recovery program. Asking for help is not a sign of weakness: it's a sign of strength. Developing coping strategies that work for you make recovery an easier road to travel.

Other professional support services include spiritual counselling, couples counselling, genetic counselling, pain clinics, long-term follow-up clinics, smoking cessation programs, and vocational rehabilitation.

Social Support

By participating in groups that share interests such as gourmet cooking, quilting, poetry reading, singing, or hiking, cancer survivors can create a circle of emotional support more as a byproduct than as their initial goal. As one canoeist says, "We're all in the same boat; we understand each other immediately." Partners and other family members of survivors have also found support either by participating in the activity or by cheering from the sidelines.

"When I joined the 'Abreast in a Boat' dragon boat team I had no idea that my husband would benefit as much as I did. He told me that being on the sidelines at the races was the best support he'd ever had. He would have never gone to a counsellor, but when he found himself standing next to other husbands who were all talking about their wives or children, he found it easy to join in. It was magical for all of us."

— Tracey, 51 years old, breast cancer, 1-year survivor

Reconnecting with a Higher Power

After treatment, some survivors embark on a search for meaning, solace, and a community with which to identify. Each of us has a unique way of expressing our spirit. Through prayer, meditation, walks in nature, walking a labyrinth, and other contemplative practices, survivors seek to honour their spirits and strengthen their connections to the divine. These connections can also be enhanced through inspirational or sacred reading, worship services, and spiritual retreats.

Some survivors begin practising yoga or Tai Chi, take up flower arranging, or begin photographing in nature with a spiritual intention. For some, this saying from spiritual writer Kahlil Gibran rings true: "To be closer to God, be closer to people." (2) You may want to join a spiritual group, connect with a spiritual advisor, or work diligently at being authentic and sincere in your relationships. Some survivors explore their deeper questions by taking a class on comparative religion or visiting a clergy member. The fundamental desire is to connect with something larger through community. Many aboriginal healing practices acknowledge that spirit is a part of everything. When we connect with each other, we connect with spirit. As we become more aware, through global interaction, of how people and cultures around the world connect with a higher power, the possibilities increase that you will find a spiritual practice that calls to you.

3. THE CREATIVE APPROACH

For many survivors, spending time exploring their creative side is the approach that most closely fits their needs. The creative approach to healing addresses the spiritual and emotional side effects of cancer.

Through the creative arts, we encounter the less verbal, less inhibited side of ourselves, which perpetually yearns to break free. People have used the creative arts for centuries to calm the mind, excite the spirit, engage the senses, focus the attention, and keep in touch with the ever-changing psyche. Creativity releases vitality, giving voice to our deepest longings. No matter what creative form you choose, you are your most authentic self when you nurture and express who you are.

"I'm energized through my photography. For me, the tactile interaction between my hands and the camera and my eyes and the scene is more than just a creative outlet. It is a means of reconnecting, a doorway to rebuilding my life."

— Meredith, 38 years old, oral cancer, 2-year survivor

Creativity is not reserved for full-time artists. The power to create exists within each of us. It lives in our imagination, and it is expressed as we go about giving unique shape and form to our everyday lives. The creative process embraces choice and chance, structure and ambiguity. In the imagination, everything is permitted.

Perhaps it's the freedom inherent in creative expression that calls to you, the chance to cast off the constraints of expectation or of an inhibiting family or culture. Or it might be the surprising richness of feeling you experience when you immerse yourself in colour, taste, fragrance, words, or sound. Follow your heart and allow yourself to try different things.

"Since I've started painting, I've begun to see things differently. I've become much more appreciative of light and shadow. I notice images I never noticed before. I've tapped into a part of me I never knew was there."

— Devon, 47 years old, colon cancer, 3-year survivor

Creativity requires absorption. When you are completely involved in a project, you are living wholly in the present. Unplugging from the external world and connecting with your inner spirit through an activity you love is very healing. Unfortunately, the Muse's voice is easily muffled by the loud call of commitments and obligations. Creating the right environment for these activities includes more than having an adequate workspace, the necessary tools and the right light. You must be willing to make the time for yourself, and to honour your art as an important part of your life.

> *"Gardening has become my creative outlet. It allows me to connect to the earth and reminds me of life, growth and the seasons. To prepare the garden and plant flowers keeps me nurturing the ground. Watering the plants every day keeps me in the moment, and when I observe the changes with each season I remember that change is just another part of the life cycle."*
> — Melinda, 54 years old, brain cancer, 4-year survivor

Whether you are a medical researcher working in a laboratory, a student writing a thesis, an amateur cook planting an herb garden or a painter working at your easel, you can be creative in what you do. Here are just a few examples of the creative exploration survivors undertake:

- **Writing:** Try journal writing, creative writing, travel writing, writing poetry, or children's stories. Write by hand or on the computer, at your desk, at the kitchen table, in a coffee shop or at the beach. Writing allows you to tell your own stories, explore your moods, or experiment with new ideas. It is a therapeutic means of self-expression.

- **Music:** Sing, chant, drum, or play whatever instrument appeals to you. Music can influence your mood. It brings you right into the present moment, and it is a pathway to the still point within. Join a choir, take singing lessons — fill your life with music.

- **Cooking:** There is nothing like the sights and smells associated with food to trigger sensory pleasure. Take cooking classes, begin a gourmet club with other couples, have a cookie exchange with friends, or plan a theme party. Modify your favourite recipes so that you can eat well and still enjoy them.

- **Visual Arts:** Painting, drawing, sculpture, woodwork, pottery: choose a medium that speaks to you and take it up. Do you like the feel of clay, the colour of paint or the grain of wood? One survivor we know makes tea pots that remind her of the issues she has faced and the support she received during treatment. She gives each pot a name: Hope, Fear, Friendship, Fragility, and so on.

It doesn't matter what you choose in the name of creativity. What matters is that you give yourself permission to experiment, to get in touch with your imagination, and to explore something that fulfills you.

4. THE CONTRIBUTING APPROACH

Contribution is about giving. It means lending a hand, sharing your time and expertise, doing good for others, caring deeply about a cause. The contributing approach to healing deals chiefly with the social and spiritual side effects of cancer.

For many survivors, the desire to contribute comes from a need to give back and to make a difference in the lives of others in their community or on the planet. All spiritual traditions emphasize the self-fulfillment that comes from serving others. Volunteer work builds personal connections and a sense of community. It helps us to see past ourselves into the larger universe. The spirit soars when we feel moved to act for another.

When we contribute to the community, our mind set shifts from an interior, contemplative focus to an external, active one. We become more grateful, more compassionate, and more loving towards others. Sheila, a 37-year-old four-year survivor of breast cancer, experienced joy when she participated in the 10K Run for the Cure: "I needed a cause that was greater than myself. I felt such a sense of accomplishment when I crossed the finish line."

Reports show that people who contribute to their communities live happier, healthier and longer lives. Doing good deepens our sense of belonging, reduces stress, and brings joy — three key health benefits. "It's better to give than to receive" is not just a moral cliché: it's proving to be a physiological boost to the immune system.

"It's my volunteer work that keeps me balanced and on track. I swear it boosts my immune system, it certainly reduces my stress, and I get so much joy from giving to others."
— Lydia, 51 years old, colorectal cancer, 2-year survivor

Contributing is an important adaptive strategy, because it supports the positive behaviour of reconnecting with yourself and with others. When you become active on behalf of a cause that you believe in, you translate caring and thinking into action. Many survivors find that the best way to approach their own healing is to participate in the healing of others. For some, this has led to a new purpose in life. Havel discovered a love of advocacy work through the volunteering he'd begun.

"I believe you need to leave the world a better place than it was when you arrived, and that is how I live each day. When I was growing up, my dad used to ask me every evening, 'Son, what good did you do for the world today?' It instilled in me a deep need to give back to others."
— Havel, 56 years old, head/neck cancer, 3-year survivor

Many survivors give back to the community by supporting other cancer patients. Sharing your experience and insights with others who are on the same journey is rewarding for both you and those you help. It's one way to ensure that something good comes from your experience. When Diane joined the Cancer Society's Reach for Recovery Program, she discovered that helping others with her type of cancer gave her a new sense of purpose. "The more you give, the more you get back," she says.

There are thousands of ways to serve the world. No one person can do it all, but each of us can create a ripple that brings greater blessings into our lives and the lives of others. By connecting to life in a tangible way, you recover a sense of control over your own life. You can start close to home: visit a sick or housebound neighbour, help at the local school or senior centre, or volunteer at your church, synagogue, mosque or temple. Moving further into your city, you can lend a hand at a food bank or an animal shelter, support the arts, or save the rivers or parks. There is always a way to be of service.

MAKING THE APPROACHES WORK: SOME SAMPLE HEALING PLANS

How do you apply your new sense of self and take charge of your recovery and ongoing healing? As a patient, you likely sought advice and permission from your doctor before you made changes in your treatments or added complementary therapies. As a survivor, you need to become your own authority on managing your recovery needs. How do you do that? By making choices and taking action on them. This is how you will develop a renewed sense of trust in yourself.

> *"I stayed with my GP for two years after my cancer treatments ended, but he didn't really help with my side effects, and I was always second-guessing him. I felt like I knew more about ovarian cancer than he did. Finally, I became assertive, started to map out my own health plan — and got a new doctor who is actually working with me."*
>
> — Miriam, 44 years old, ovarian cancer, 3-year survivor

Healing is a journey unique to each individual. However, it's never easy to know where to begin. To guide you, we have provided you with four samples of survivors' Healing Plans. Each plan focuses on one or more of the four approaches presented in this chapter. Each identifies both the survivor's intentions and the specific actions he or she plans to take to fulfill them.

Kevin: The Physical Approach

Kevin was a 26-year-old university student on spring break when he first discovered his melanoma. His treatment included surgery and the use of an experimental drug. His relationship with his girlfriend is solid, and in his spare time he loves playing guitar and writing songs. He had never paid much attention to his health before the cancer, but now, one month after his treatment ended, his primary healing approach is physical, aimed at restoring and strengthening his body.

KEVIN'S HEALING PLAN

I want to focus my healing efforts on ... *my physical health.*

INTENTIONS	ACTIONS
1. To improve my immune system	1. Start dietary changes — eliminate sugar, caffeine and alcohol, and add one more fruit and/or vegetable to each meal.
	2. Begin taking anti-oxidant vitamins and supplements.
	3. Work with a traditional Chinese medicine doctor.
2. To improve my physical strength and increase my energy	1. Exercise in gym 3x/week for 45 minutes; begin weight-training, stretching and 15 minutes of aerobics.
	2. Go to bed by 10:00 p.m. to get eight hours of sleep.

Betty: The Creative Approach

Betty is a 52-year-old wife and mother who runs an active household with three teenaged children, as well as working part-time from her home as a bookkeeper. She has always been physically active and eats a well-balanced diet. Her treatment for breast cancer included surgery, chemotherapy and radiation therapy. Now, four months later, she still feels fragmented, has low energy, and lacks confidence in her future. She has always been interested in painting but has never made time to look into it. Her primary goal is to spend more time alone, exploring her feelings and igniting her healing energies through pursuing art.

BETTY'S HEALING PLAN

I want to focus my healing efforts on ... *rekindling my passion and sense of purpose through creativity.*

INTENTIONS	ACTIONS
1. To reconnect with myself through art	1. Daily journal writing to explore feelings.
	2. Make time to paint 3x/week.
	3. Take daily walks with my dog by the ocean to stimulate my creative spirit.

Julian: The Connected Approach

Julian is a 44-year-old, one-year survivor of lymphoma. His treatment included chemotherapy and radiation. He works long hours in the small business he owns and has been married for sixteen years with two children. Julian grew up in a very religious family but left the church when he moved away from home after high school. He is a physically active man who volunteers in his community by coaching his younger son's soccer team, and he and his wife have a wide social circle. However, since his cancer he has been fluctuating between periods of restlessness, agitation and depression. He wants to return to a place of worship but isn't sure which one. In his plan, he is choosing to focus on addressing his emotional volatility, connecting with his family and rekindling his religious faith.

JULIAN'S HEALING PLAN

I want to focus my healing efforts on ... *connecting with my emotions, with my family, and with God.*

INTENTIONS	ACTIONS
1. To address my emotional volatility and mood swings	1. See a psychiatrist or counsellor. 2. Work for 30 minutes each day in the garden.
2. To spend more time with my family	1. Be home for dinner 4x / week. 2. Spend some alone time with each son.
3. To find a church and become an active member	1. Meet with the clergy of three local churches, attend services, meet members of the congregation and make a commitment to join one.

Lorna: A Mixed Approach

Lorna is a 37-year-old, nine-month survivor of colorectal cancer. Her treatment included surgery resulting in a colostomy and nerve damage that left her with chronic pain and sexual dysfunction. Her mother and husband have been her primary supports in helping her to deal with her losses, which included giving up the job she loved but could no longer work at due to the long hours of standing. In her plan, she chooses to deal with the physical and emotional issues she's experiencing.

LORNA'S HEALING PLAN

I want to focus my healing efforts on ... *physical healing and connecting with others to get the support I need.*

INTENTIONS	ACTIONS
1. To start a pain management regime	1. Get a referral from my GP to a pain specialist.
	2. Investigate the local pain clinic.
2. To improve my body image	1. Attend a yoga class 3x/week.
	2. Speak with a sexuality counsellor.
3. To make peace with my losses	1. Join a "Living with Loss" support group.
	2. Start a grief journal.

CREATING YOUR OWN HEALING PLAN

Once you have decided which aspect of your health to focus on, it is time to set some healing goals that are both reasonable and attainable. A central premise of this book is that the physical, emotional, spiritual and social aspects of our health are inseparable: we can't truly heal one part of ourselves without healing the others. Any positive step that you take towards healing will have a ripple effect. One small step can make a big difference.

Your healing plan will provide a means of sorting through your choices and then of clarifying your intentions. While we encourage you to set healing intentions that encompass all aspects of your life, you should begin where you can. For some survivors, it is enough at first to create a daily routine that includes small but achievable changes: adding two vegetables to your diet, setting aside a brief period each day for rest or quiet time, or completing your daily practices.

Start with a fresh page in your recovery journal for your Healing Plan. As you fill it in, think about where you would like to focus your healing efforts. Your intentions will depend to a large extent on when your treatments ended. Try not to compare yourself with others or your healing choices with those of anyone else. Take into consideration your current state of health, including any day-to-day fluctuations in energy and both physical and emotional side effects. Review your Self Scans and your list of energy builders and drainers. Think about your strengths, your limitations, the positive changes you have already made and the losses you have yet to grieve. What is currently motivating you to action? Are your healing goals based on fear — keeping the cancer at bay — or on a desire to live well?

The Taoist philosopher Lao-Tzu said, "A journey of 1,000 miles begins with a single step." (3) Now is the time to take your first step in reclaiming your health and beginning the healing journey.

Ask yourself:

- Where do I want to focus my healing efforts? Which of the four healing approaches — physical, connected, creative, or contributing — feels right for me? Do I want to take a combination approach instead?
- What are my healing intentions?
- Which behaviours or specific actions will help me achieve my desired results?

INTENTIONS	ACTIONS
MY HEALING PLAN I want to focus my healing efforts on:	
1.	1. 2.
2.	1. 2.
3.	1. 2.
4.	1. 2.
5.	1. 2.

TAKING THE NEXT STEP

One of the biggest steps on your healing journey is simply deciding which direction to take. By clarifying your intentions and your actions, you have stepped boldly forward.

You're now at the point where, as they say, the rubber meets the road. You need to put your Healing Plan into motion, and this requires action. Before you begin to implement your desired changes, though, look at how you can maximize your chances for success.

CHAPTER ELEVEN

Actualizing Your Healing Plan

"I knew I needed to change my old patterns and behaviours; I'd stayed there long enough. I was open to trying lots of new activities, which motivated me to explore other areas of my life that needed healing. Once I decided to change my mindset, my options were endless."

— Zeina, 41 years old, breast cancer, 1-year survivor

"I always thought what I needed was to take a big leap, but in truth I need to choose a few small steps and commit to doing them. I am a good one for big leaps, but not so good at little steps. In the past I had trouble committing to the things I knew I had to do. Now I try to keep focused on the small but necessary goals."

— Marvin, 56 years old, lung cancer, 2-year survivor

Now that you have identified the actions you need to take in your Healing Plan, you'll be eager to get started. When you choose one action over another, you are taking charge of change and recovering your sense of control. This is in direct contrast to the unpredictable and involuntary changes that may have come with your cancer.

It is through action that we strengthen our bodies, renew our spirits, and bring joy into our lives. It is in the *doing* of something that learning and growth occur. Adopting a can-do, ready-for-action attitude will assist you through this phase of your recovery process. But before you press on with the Healing Plan you've designed, it's a good idea to consider the obstacles you might encounter. That way, you'll be prepared to meet them when they arise.

POTENTIAL OBSTACLES

It's important to acknowledge that you will likely encounter some form of resistance — internal or external — to your personal healing goals. Thinking ahead about who or what may block your path toward change and being prepared with strategies to defy this resistance will dramatically increase your chances of success. Let's look at the two most predictable obstacles: the pull of the status quo and the persistence of old habits. Both are rooted in a desire for the familiar; the status quo represents the pressure others place upon you to remain the same, while old habits are the corresponding internal pressure to return to the known.

The Pull of Status Quo

Human beings are self-regulating systems, and all such systems are characterized by a pull to maintain equilibrium. In biology, this is called *homeostasis,* and it applies to our psychological states, our social behaviour, and our physical functioning. Each of us exists within a number of systems: we come from one family system, usually live later in another, and work and play in still others. Within each system there are roles and expectations. Some of these serve our growth and development, and some do not. The balancing forces of homeostasis are neither good nor bad, but they can prevent you from pursuing new opportunities by encouraging you to return to the status quo.

For survivors, the pressure other people put on you to return to your old self is one example. Don't be surprised if the people you love start subtly or openly to undermine your attempts at change. They do not wish you harm; it is just homeostasis at work.

> *"Right after treatment ended, I wanted to get back in shape. The people I used to work out with kept asking me why I didn't come anymore. The truth is, I had my eye on a yoga class. That's what appealed to me. 'Yoga!' they laughed. 'You won't break a sweat with yoga.'"*
>
> — Samira, 34 years old, lymphoma, 5-month survivor

The Persistence of Old Habits

It is ironic that change is the one constant in our lives, and yet the act of changing is so hard. Ingrained habits can put up resistance that brings us to a standstill. A *habit* is a tendency to act in a certain way, a pattern of behaviour acquired by frequent repetition that can become involuntary. We fall into or call upon ingrained habits when we go on automatic pilot, whether in the ways we brush our teeth or the route we take home from work. When things are going smoothly, there is little incentive to change old habits or look for better ways to do things. As the saying goes, "If it ain't broke, don't fix it."

However, the ambiguity and uncertainty triggered by your post-cancer transition provide a positive impetus to review, renew or start over. Pursuing your Healing Plan will require you first to become aware of your old habits, then to commit to replacing those that aren't helping you with healthy, life-affirming new ones. The good news is that we can change our habits. But to break undesirable habits and form new ones takes both time and frequent repetition.

ENSURING SUCCESS

To ensure success, you will need to build support from the family members and friends who will be most affected by your plans. Let those close to you know about your Healing Plan. If family and friends are unaware of your healing intentions, they can unknowingly become obstacles. Support from others gives you the strength to pursue your goals through adversity, cynicism, self-doubt, apathy and resignation. It also helps you keep perspective and maintain balance. But not all support is the same. It's important to determine what kind you need.

Examples of different types of support persons include those who:

- are physically present
- listen without judgment
- give constructive feedback
- encourage and motivate you
- validate your goals
- love you
- provide a distraction for you

- give physical, tangible help
- offer suggestions and advice
- provide information
- are your cheerleaders

Gathering allies can make the difference between succeeding with your Healing Plan and struggling with it. Even when your desire is strong, there are days when you'll need your support people to help you through a difficult day.

Remember, too, that your needs can change over time. As you take action, you will find yourself developing more confidence and resourcefulness. You may find you require less of one kind of support but more of another as you move closer to achieving your recovery goals. Don't be afraid to change your support people as you need to, depending on your progress, new insights, and change in direction.

TOOLS TO HELP YOU ACTUALIZE YOUR PLAN

Clarifying your intentions may have helped you see discrepancies between your current level of recovery and where you'd like to be. It's this awareness that motivates you to take action. The drive to achieve your goals, coupled with a clear plan about how to do it readies you to pursue change. It is time to switch off the autopilot and proceed by manual control towards the healing you desire. Start by copying down in your recovery journal the action(s) you chose in the Healing Plan you designed in Chapter 10. Then ask yourself: What do I need to do to pursue my healing goals?

For each action you chose, you will want to:

- **Clarify potential obstacles** (lack of time, support, money, etc.): what or who might keep you from achieving your goal?

- **Identify your support system**: who will you ask, and for what kind of help? Make a list of the people you can depend on to help you achieve your plan. This may include family, friends, neighbours, co-workers, church members, health care providers and other survivors.

- **Develop strategies**: what might you use to overcome the obstacles you've identified? Hiring a babysitter, asking a friend to check in regularly, signing up for a weekly class or joining a group activity others expect you to attend are just a few examples.

COMMIT TO ACT

We are all motivated to do what is important to us. Hence, there must be a connection between your Healing Plan and the sincerity of your promise to yourself to pursue it. Action is fuelled by commitment. Commitment is the hardest step towards living well, though, because it means staying on target even when other things may be depleting your energy.

> *"When I get depressed, angry, or fearful, I stay home and watch videos and wait for the feelings to pass. Exercise would be good for me, but I don't go because I tell myself my breathing will become a problem. The truth is I'm lazy, and it takes energy to go out and do something. I want to change my life, but I can't seem to make the commitment, even to myself."*
> — Barbara, 51 years old, lung cancer, 2-year survivor

Commitment is fragile, and it requires continual care. It involves focus, discipline and a large dose of persistence. But the rewards of making a commitment are numerous. Taking action reduces fear, unleashes imagination and creativity, and enhances your quality of life.

> *"I had to commit, and I mean really commit, to respecting myself and honouring my healing needs. For me, art was the doorway to rebuilding my life. It became more than a frivolous hobby; it was what gave me new direction."*
> — Hector, 43 years old, lymphoma, 3-year survivor

You may be eager to change and try new things. At the same time, you feel insecure, incompetent, and frightened. Even in your darkest hour, can you commit to doing one thing you feel good about, whether it is joining a support group, taking a creative writing class, or volunteering for a cause close to your heart? Fatigue, pain, and depression can easily shut you down, so take the rest you need, and make sure you and your health care team are dealing with your side effects in an effective way. As you move forward into action, do everything you can to stay on your Healing Plan.

TAKE ACTION

There is risk in action. Until you act, there is hope and possibility. When you act on those possibilities, you are faced with reality. Often reality will support your hopes. Sometimes it may even exceed them. We have all had the experience, too, of attempting an action that seems filled with possibility only to discover that the reality falls short of our expectations.

There are times for thought and for planning, and both are important. But at some points in your life you must act despite your fears and doubts. Waiting for the right conditions to appear — for the kids to leave home, for retirement — is a luxury you now realize you can't afford. Once you've decided to act, muster your resolve and run with it.

May the creed of the Scottish Himalayan Expedition, written by W.N. Murray, inspire you as you move forward in your recovery:

> *Until one is committed, there is hesitancy,*
> *The chance to draw back, always ineffectiveness.*
> *Concerning all acts of initiative and creation*
> *There is one elemental truth, the ignorance of which*
> *Kills countless ideas and splendid plans:*
> *The moment one definitely commits oneself,*
> *Then Providence moves, too.*
> *All sort of things occur to help one that would otherwise never have occurred.*
> *A whole stream of events issues from the decision,*
> *Raising in one's favour all manner of unforeseen incidents and*
> *Meetings and material assistance,*
> *Which no man could have dreamed would have come his way.* (1)

CHAPTER TWELVE

Exploring Possibility

"I'd been given a second chance at life, and I grabbed it. I decided it was time to do something with my life, not just in my life."

— Walter, 45 years old, lymphoma, 3-year survivor

"I had time to reassess what was truly important to me, and I found most things were intact. I believed in the values I had been taught. I had my relationships in order. It was reassuring to know I was living the life I wanted to live."

— Jeannette, 48 years old, lung cancer, 1-year survivor

Congratulations — you've designed your Healing Plan and begun acting on it. You are determined to take charge of your life. Yet, as you move steadily forward, things will be shifting and evolving, often in more ways than you could have anticipated. New questions will likely emerge. As your healing progresses, you'll want to take some time to sit back and dream, to see what big picture is emerging as the edges of your puzzle take shape.

During the first few months of recovery, many survivors are grateful just to be alive, and they find it difficult to think beyond the present day. Some survivors are happy to have more time to continue the life they've been leading. But others view their illness as a wake-up call. They find themselves engaged in a serious reappraisal of their lives, identifying areas where they feel things have become derailed. For some people, the wake-up call means release from a job, a marriage, and or a plan other people have held for them. Others begin reconsidering lost desires, long-held hopes and newly imagined dreams. All survivors face a challenging question: *Now that I didn't die, how will I choose to live?*

SEEK AND YOU WILL FIND

The process of Discovery is rooted in exploration. Exploration is one of the few things you can do without risk of failure, since mining the possibilities is your only goal. During treatment, your primary goal was survival. Your recovery period is the time for saying "yes" to life, for pursuing opportunities that will move you closer to feeling whole.

To become an adventurer in your own life — despite your fear or anxiety — you must approach new possibilities with openness, curiosity and courage. This may sound daunting. *What do I want?* you may be asking yourself. It's not always easy to know. You have to listen for that small voice that speaks from your core self. Daily life makes a lot of noise. So does your inner critic, who is quite prepared to shoot down new ideas as soon as you have them, with a hundred reasons why *You can't do that!*

The poet Emily Dickinson wrote, "I dwell in Possibility ..." (1) Living with that mindset means allowing yourself to be inquisitive, to stretch beyond what you already know, even beyond what you or others might think impossible. *Are you living the life you want to live?* If you're not sure, or if you feel a nagging desire to set goals that transcend day-to-day survival, now is the time to do something about it.

There is an old saying: "How we spend our days is how we spend our lives." Once you awaken to the voice of your heart, you may find your life moving in directions you never dreamed possible. This is where courage comes in. The root of courage is "coeur," which means heart. It takes courage to follow your heart and pursue your passion.

To respond to the call of life means to take more risks, to trust in yourself. Rather than putting a lid on the possibilities that present themselves during your recovery, take a leap of faith and give yourself a second chance.

"It was a defining moment when I decided to leave my job as a school teacher and begin concentrating on opening my own business as an educational consultant. It gave me many new freedoms, a sense of accomplishment and in the end a better pay cheque. But most importantly, it allowed me to live the way I wanted to live."

— Jeff, 48 years old, lymphoma, 4-year survivor

A SECOND CHANCE

As a survivor of cancer, you now have a second chance at life. Cancer may turn out to be the catalyst you needed to pursue new dreams or make changes you've wanted to make for a long time. As your recovery progresses, your priorities often shift. What was once pressing may no longer be so, while other things claim new urgency. You need to keep asking yourself, *What's important to me, and what isn't? What do I need to hold onto, and what do I choose to let go of?*

Making new choices gives you a second chance to live well. This may involve renewing your sense of purpose and recommitting to your loved ones. Or it may mean shaking your life up, even starting over. For some people, this second chance brings the opportunity to "go big," to make the kinds of changes that before cancer they have only dreamed about. Second chances come along rarely. You can respond with a new awareness, an attitude shift, a softening of old ways, or a monumental life change.

"Before the cancer I was so caught up in the busyness of my life. Now if my husband calls and asks if I want to take a drive and see the new goslings in the lake, I drop everything and go. The laundry and cooking can wait."

— Deirdre, 53 years old, lung cancer, 3-year survivor

WHOSE PERMISSION DO YOU NEED?

As you pursue your Healing Plan, can you give yourself permission to explore? Can you allow yourself to let go and try something new? The process can be frightening, but it is also exciting, and only you can make it happen.

"After treatment ended, I felt like I was alone in the woods without a flashlight. I had to keep reminding myself, 'Odette, let go. Cast off the straitjacket of the past. Your cancer could come back, so get on with what you want.' Nobody else was going to give that permission to me. I had to give it to myself."

— Odette, 34 years old, cervical cancer, 10-month survivor

Now is the time to give yourself permission to do what you need to do, whether it's taking a long walks on the beach or embarking on a new career. This may be difficult. In balancing your needs with the needs of loved ones, you will inevitably encounter tension and competing desires.

"Sometimes when I'm meditating or going to an acting class, I feel guilty because I think I should be doing the ironing or cleaning the house. I'm not comfortable spending the time on myself when I know how much there is to do for my family."

— Alicia, 37 years old, lymphoma, 15-month survivor

But re-embracing life after nearly losing it also brings new insight and confidence. Many survivors realize they must overcome their feelings of helplessness and say "no" to energy drainers, "yes" to the things they truly enjoy.

"I allow myself to go to the movies in the afternoon, to enjoy long chess games with my neighbour, and to read late into the night when I've got a great book. After all, who knows how much time I have left?"

— Kirk, 62 years old, prostate cancer, 1-year survivor

Your greatest calling is to be your most authentic self, whether or not that conforms to other people's ideas of what's nice or right. This means restructuring your life so that, at some point every day, you take priority.

"I finally decided to put myself at the top of the list. I've been meeting everyone else's needs for quite a while now. Every day before my husband and children get up I jump out of bed, make myself some tea and then write children's stories. I always wanted to be a writer but never thought

I'd be any good. Now I write for me first. We'll see if the publisher likes
it later."

— Joan, 50 years old, breast cancer, 2-year survivor

ENVISIONING THE LIFE YOU WANT TO LIVE

It's hard to jump into living the life you want to live without a clear picture of what that looks like. Having a vision of what you want helps you to see clearly where you are going. It can be a beacon in times of chaos, giving you a sense of control by providing direction. Your vision of the life you want can help you develop a self-confidence that comes from believing in your ability to take charge. It can guide your choices and give you a sense of stability. It helps you to decide where you want to spend your time and your energy.

Change does not have to happen on a grand scale for it to be profound. Your vision might consist of a few small but significant changes that better align your external life with your authentic self. What's important is that the picture you create is meaningful to you.

"My vision of living well meant doing a few very specific things: taking
time out when I was tired; keeping in touch with friends who were impor-
tant to me; being kind to others; being generous; and supporting others
living with cancer."

— Bernadette, 58 years old, ovarian cancer, 2-year survivor

A personal vision is a clear, compelling view of a desired future. Larger than a goal and more achievable than a fantasy, a vision is a picture of where you want to go and what you will be like when you get there. Your vision of tomorrow can help you get through the trials of today and withstand the negative pull of the past.

DARE TO SEE YOURSELF LIVING WELL

The writer Henry David Thoreau encourages us to go confidently in the direction of our dreams and live the lives we've imagined. (2) Your vision of living well is your path to wholeness after cancer. It will inspire you to get moving again.

Be patient with yourself — this is just the beginning. As you follow the concrete actions your Healing Plan sets out, pay attention to what is nudging you on a deeper level. Every so often, take the time to close your eyes and let yourself dream. Relax, take a few deep breaths, let go of the tension in your body and picture yourself living vibrantly. Let your mind wander without restrictions. We encourage you to unlock the flood gates of possibility and allow yourself to really see the person you want to be. What do you see yourself doing? How do you feel? What images come to mind? Use this technique as often you want. It's simple, it doesn't cost anything, and the results can be life changing.

YOUR WILD AND PRECIOUS LIFE

When you look back on your life, you do not want to be haunted by regrets — unexplored possibilities or unfinished business. Some survivors grieve the doors of opportunity that cancer has slammed shut. But every time one door shuts, another opens.

It takes time and commitment to figure out what you really want. Operating from a place of possibility, though, you can create the life you choose. In her poem "The Summer Day" Mary Oliver expresses the sentiment beautifully:

> *Doesn't everything die at last, and too soon?*
> *Tell me, what is it you plan to do*
> *with your one wild and precious life?* (3)

Attentive Walking

As you walk, see whether you catch your thoughts drifting to old dreams or abandoned desires. Observe where these thoughts take you. Notice what messages your heart sends you. Many artists and writers claim they get their best ideas while walking. Then gently bring your attention back to the present moment. *Just keep walking.*

The Five-Question Check-In

From time to time, after you complete the five-question check-in, look back over your previous answers to see whether you can recognize any patterns or recurring themes. Your deepest yearnings may be showing up. Be aware of any possibilities presenting themselves to you and allow yourself to explore whatever arises. Your answers to the daily questions will give you clues about which aspects of yourself are calling out and which need more attention.

CHAPTER THIRTEEN

Re-Evaluating
Your Healing Plan

"My plan is working. I'm managing my fatigue with the help of my doctor and a nutritionist, and I'm walking every day. I can finally see the fog lifting."

— Maurice, 31 years old, testicular cancer, 6-month survivor

"I was off and running with my new eating and exercise schedule. I incorporated fitness into my daily routine and drastically changed my diet. I also joined the local community centre's mentorship program for disadvantaged children. But soon I couldn't keep up with my original plan; I was overextended in every direction. I had to re-evaluate and make new choices, ones that keep me healthy but weren't overwhelming my day."

— Florence, 48 years old, cervical cancer, 9-month survivor

Once you've spent time following your Healing Plan, you may realize that some of your choices need altering. Maybe your plan has pushed you to take more risks than you're ready for. Maybe you don't feel challenged enough. Once you've decided on a healing approach and begun to make changes in your life, it's crucial to step back periodically to review what's working and what isn't. Taking the time to evaluate what you're doing is as important as accomplishing the tasks themselves. Are you proceeding in the direction you had hoped? Are your investments of time and energy in new pursuits paying off? Do the results match your intentions? Reviewing, assessing, and readjusting are essential aspects of the Discovery Phase of recovery.

Your needs and desires will change as your recovery progresses. Your perspective will change too. New information will come to light. Your circumstances may shift. Perhaps you've discovered that, thanks to your health care team, your side effects have diminished and you can resume an activity you'd written off as impossible six months ago. Perhaps a new drug has come onto the market. Perhaps your situation at work has changed. To be effective, your Healing Plan will need to keep pace with the constant flux of your life.

FINE-TUNING YOUR PLAN

Before you make any changes to your Healing Plan, you will want to review your original healing intentions and consider to what degree your actions have helped you achieve the desired results. Be honest with yourself. Pay attention to your feelings and intuitions. You may find that despite your clear intention to calm your anxiety by attending meditation sessions, you are simply not going. Pilates may be the hot new exercise, but you may find it as dull as watching paint dry.

While there is no set time rule, we recommend that you review your Healing Plan every four to six weeks for as long as you need to. Each time you re-evaluate, you will make one of three discoveries:

- **It's a go**: your plan is working fine, and you are making progress.
- **Take a step back**: your plan does not seem to be working well, and you are frustrated.
- **Add to your plan**: your original plan no longer seems challenging enough.

Let's look again at the sample Healing Plans we outlined in Chapter 10, this time to see what happened when the four survivors re-examined their choices.

It's a Go!

Remember Kevin, the university student who chose a physical approach to healing? With the changes he planned to make to his diet and exercise regime, Kevin intended to improve his immune system and to increase both his energy and his physical strength.

After two months of sticking to his plan, Kevin noticed a marked improvement in the way he was feeling. His fatigue had diminished, he had lost some weight and gained back muscle, and he particularly enjoyed the work he was doing with the Chinese medicine doctor. Evaluating the results of his plan confirmed to Kevin that he was on the right track. He decided to continue his regime and planned another evaluation in two months' time.

Take a Step Back

Betty was the mother and part-time bookkeeper who chose the creative approach to healing. She had planned to write in her journal every day, to walk her dog daily by the ocean and to find time to paint three times a week.

Betty, however, had three teenaged children, all of whom needed her time and attention. Her plan of painting three times a week soon dwindled to two, then one, then none at all. Walking the dog became the old chore it used to be, because she rarely had time to get down to the beach.

After six weeks, Betty was frustrated. She suspected she was unconsciously sabotaging her Healing Plan. To compound things, she had had to take on some new clients to compensate for a cutback in her husband's work hours. She felt stressed and disappointed and wondered whether she had expected too much of herself. For these reasons, she decided to join a support group, where she befriended another breast cancer survivor who became a great ally. With her new friend's encouragement, Betty enrolled in a painting class that motivated her to show up at the canvas at least once a week. She modified her Healing Plan to balance her healing needs with family and time demands and felt she had gained an appreciation of the obstacles that can get in the way of even the most desired change.

Add to Your Plan

Lorna was the survivor whose Healing Plan was geared to dealing with both physical healing and a sense of emotional loss. Six months after initiating her plan, Lorna was happy with the results she was seeing. Her pain had decreased substantially. She was feeling better about her body image and had gained strength and confidence from working with a sexuality counsellor and attending yoga classes. Through her support group, she was beginning to deal with her grief. Lorna was content to continue working with her current Healing Plan, but she also felt she needed more joy and creativity in her life. Since she had always loved to sing, she decided to join a choir at the local community center, and she added this activity to her plan.

Julian was the businessman who wanted to reconnect with his feelings, his family, and his faith. After investigating several churches in his area, he decided to join the United Church. As he began attending services, Julian discovered his interest in spirituality was much deeper than he had realized. One year after designing his original Healing Plan, he had become so excited about this discovery that he decided to enrol part-time at the university to do graduate work in religious studies, with the goal of becoming a minister.

STAY FLEXIBLE

Kevin, Betty, Lorna, and Julian all found it useful to re-evaluate their Healing Plans. Kevin learned he was still on track. The others made new choices. When you're re-assessing your own Healing Plan, you'll want to be careful not to compare your recovery to anyone else's. Your goal is to progress at a pace that is right for you.

Your re-evaluation will provide you with new information, and with that comes the possibility of change. Keep an open and flexible attitude towards the things you try. Although you should not see your Healing Plan at any stage as set in stone, remember that it takes 21 days of consistently performing a new behaviour before it becomes a habit. If something doesn't work after you've given it a good shot, don't be afraid to change your mind and try a new idea. Detours are as much a part of life as the direct route. In her book *When Life Changes or You Wish It Would*, Carol Adrienne encourages us: "Life is rich with false starts, regressions, retractions, impulsive moves, first impressions, calculated waiting and panicked What have I dones? This is all part of the creative flow of life — to be enjoyed, rejoiced in and wondered at." (1)

WHAT CAN TAKE YOU OFF THE HEALING PATH?

Even the most committed person can stumble, and the best plans can get derailed. Sometimes, despite the best intentions and a good Healing Plan, you can find yourself slipping back into old habits, even ones that do not serve you. Slipping often starts slyly. For example, you don't keep your volunteer commitment on Tuesday for a specific reason. But then you find yourself cancelling the following week too, because "something came up." It's not long before your resolve starts to weaken and you're not volunteering any longer.

No forward movement is sustainable unless you identify and understand what pushes you back. As we have outlined in Chapter 11, the pull of old habits and the status quo are two common forms of resistance, but there are other forces that can hinder your progress. Here's a brief list of some of the challenges survivors face:

- **A refusal to listen to your inner voice.** You find yourself denying what your inner voice is telling you about where you need to be or what you need to do for yourself. *I know I should make some changes to my lifestyle, but now just doesn't seem like the right time.*

- **Guilt and obligations** from relationships and other social pressures like child-care responsibilities, taking care of elderly parents, work, etc. *There's only so much time in a day. I know I should take care of myself, but everyone needs me. I have to go back to being the person they want me to be.*

- **Real-life stressors** such as illness in the family, loss of a job, financial concerns, etc. *I really want to start painting, but being a single parent with crazy work hours, I don't feel I can justify taking the time or spending the money on an art class.*

- **Doubt and lack of trust.** The "what if?" questions. *What if Chinese medicine doesn't work? What if I can't commit to my plan?*

- **Lack of commitment.** *I want to walk four times a week, but somehow I never get around to it.*

- **Fear.** A fear of failure: a fear of success. *I'm not sure I'd be any good at going to the gym so I just stay home. I'm afraid I'll lose my job if I don't agree to work overtime. I'm afraid my marriage will fall apart if I start asking for what I want.*

- **Over-confidence.** *Everything is going to be fine; it will all take care of itself. I don't need to do anything to change my life. I don't need help from anyone.*

- **Lack of time.** An unwillingness to make yourself a priority in your own life. *I try to fit meditation into my schedule, but I'm so busy; I always have a million things to do.*

- **Loss of hope.** *What's the use in trying anything? The cancer will just come back. What I do makes no difference. Nothing is going to change.*

- **Impatience.** Change isn't happening quickly enough for you. *It's been three weeks since I changed my lifestyle and I don't feel any better.*

- **Lack of support.** *I was counting on my neighbour to baby-sit for me twice a week while I went to the local lap pool, but now she's started a new job and can't do it.*

Know this: you *will* run into obstacles. When it happens, don't get discouraged or allow these roadblocks to dissuade you from your goals. Greet the obstacles, then get ready to negotiate.

DEVELOPING EFFECTIVE STRATEGIES

Strategies provide you with tangible steps you can take even when your willpower or energy falter. They allow you to sustain momentum and achieve results even when you do not feel motivated. It must be said, however, that if you have chosen actions for your Healing Plan that correspond with your true desires, these actions often carry their own motivation: they make you happy. If you are not feeling satisfied, you might have to take a second look at your choices and ask yourself whether they really stem from your authentic self.

Rarely are there perfect solutions for our problems. We can usually come up with *viable* solutions, though. Some will require more experimentation or compromise than others. Here are some strategies you might consider for getting yourself back on the healing path. They do not appear in any particular order. Choose the one — or several — that best suits your needs.

Create a Diversion

There are times when we need to step back in order to gain perspective. If frustration sets in, it might mean you have been trying too hard to make something happen in a certain way. Take a break. Have a cup of tea, watch a movie, hit some golf balls, or take a candlelit bath. Choose an activity you love that will distract you for a little while from taking charge of change.

Fresh eyes and new energy do wonders for decision-making. Taking a break buys you some time and gives you space to take a deep breath. Afterwards, you will be in a better position to decide whether or not to pursue the same course of action. However, a word of warning: don't be too quick to judge that something isn't working or to replace one goal with another. Frustrations are to be expected when you are attempting to change old habits or introduce new behaviours. Try to be patient, and remember the three-week rule for forming new habits.

Learn from the Past

When you consider your past with an open mind and a soft heart, you might discover you've been through challenging situations before, facing obstacles that seemed insurmountable at the time. Some of those situations may have triggered a crisis. Some may have been turning points for you, while others simply provided tough lessons. You may have adapted to some adversities and recovered quickly. Others took longer, and you required support to get through them.

Your resilience is enhanced when you mine the rich experiences of your past. You may have been down this road before. What worked last time? What didn't? Can you use past transitions to help you navigate the present one?

Journal writing is a helpful exercise for this strategy. Just sit down and write. No one will read what you've written except you. Let your hand move across the page without taking time to evaluate what you are writing until you're done. Explore where you've been in your life without judgment, negativity, or guilt. Often the answers we seek are within.

Follow Your Positive Energy

Positive energy comes from participating in activities that stimulate you, release you from stress, or bring you joy. It also comes from holding thoughts of hope, love, compassion, forgiveness, and trust. When you draw on your positive energy, you affirm your wholeness and create a sense of well-being. Many survivors access positive feelings by tapping into their connection to the divine or using contemplative practices such as meditation or prayer. Others are rejuvenated through their relationships or some form of creative expression. Do your homework. Gather suggestions from other survivors, from websites and cancer newsletters, from books and health care practitioners. Find the resources that will work for you. Move towards what attracts or inspires you.

Here are some ideas from other survivors:

- **Find a good role model.** Look around for someone who inspires you to action, someone you believe has made good choices in overcoming adversity.

- **Learn what "no" means.** Sometimes saying no is a good way to set limits, but sometimes it is a sign that you're stuck in a rut. Perhaps this is the time to say "yes" instead.

- **Pamper yourself.** Find small or large ways to bring more pleasure into your life. Buy your favourite kind of tea, put fresh flowers in your bedroom, cozy up with a good book, or schedule a relaxing massage. Be kind to yourself.

- **Create an inspiring motto** for yourself and tape it to your computer or your refrigerator door.

The bottom line? Change what you can. Live with the things you can't change. Always move forward.

Trust Yourself

Sometimes the changes that accompany cancer are so intense that all you can do is hope everything will eventually be okay. Initially, most survivors turn to their doctors and other members of their health care team for reassurance. They look to those with more knowledge and authority than themselves. This is not surprising; we are socially and culturally trained to go outside ourselves for answers. But although you may choose to follow the advice of others, the final authority always remains with you. No one else can choose your direction. No one else knows how best to meet your unique conditions for healing.

Believe in the path you've chosen to follow and in yourself. No one will take you seriously if your commitment is lukewarm. When you own your vision emphatically, it becomes yours. Say it out loud to yourself and to others. Stand up for yourself and your needs and desires. Allow your body to speak. Let it tell you whether or not you are okay. Accept that you will feel some anxiety or fear when you take charge of your own healthy choices. Fear and doubt are not problems to be solved, but rather forces to be understood.

In learning to trust yourself again, you may need to begin with the physical results: what you can see.

"I started observing and recording how the different actions I took affected my pain. One surprising discovery after a physiotherapy appointment was that although my pain had only been reduced slightly, the range of motion in my arm was greatly improved. Slowly but surely I began to see results."
— Maureen, 36 years old, breast cancer, 3-month survivor

A major impediment to trusting yourself might be the negative beliefs that whisper you are not worth the time and trouble it takes to pursue the life you want. Replace these self-sabotaging thoughts with more rational ones. When the naysayers either within you or around you start to speak, pick powerful responses that will work for you. Try these:

- I choose what's right for me.
- I need to do this for myself.
- Hey, I just faced death. What am I waiting for?
- If I don't do it now, then when?

Forgive Yourself

Everybody trips. Be gentle with yourself when it happens to you. Every setback is an opportunity for learning something new, about either yourself or your circumstances. Often we learn more from our setbacks than from our successes. Perhaps the most important skill we acquire is to pick ourselves up, dust off, and try again. But persistence must be accompanied by the willingness to forgive yourself when you fall. When you forgive yourself for a setback, you are freeing yourself from self-criticism or blame. You are demonstrating trust in your own ability to start again with renewed energy and optimism.

Adapt and Adjust

When you make changes that integrate the essential lessons of your experience, you are making an adaptive response. To adapt is to make adjustments. There is no one magical adaptive strategy. Trust in your ability to know which strategy will work for you. Eventually, your behaviour will fall in line with your beliefs. When that happens, you will be "walking your talk," allowing your actions to express your authentic self. Commit yourself to living each day as fully and joyfully as you can.

RE-COMMITMENT: ONE STEP AT A TIME

Re-evaluating your Healing Plan allows you to re-examine where you want to put your energy, and to discard issues and actions that are not a current priority. Keeping the commitments you make to yourself means honouring them with the same integrity you use when you give your word to a dear friend. Some days, this is easier said than done. Most of us lead busy but undisciplined lives, and often it takes a crisis to make us stop and reflect. For many survivors, cancer was that crisis. Yet it still takes remarkable courage to cut back and channel your resources into only a few areas. There may be days when you feel apathetic about carrying out your daily activities, let alone following your Healing Plan.

In his book *Laws of the Spirit*, Dan Millman writes, "People rarely ever fail; they only stop trying." He reminds us, "Lasting progress doesn't happen in a few dramatic moments, but hour by hour, day by day. As time passes every process includes repairs: the road to happiness is always under construction." (2)

Obstacles to change can slow you down, even require you to detour, but they need not stop you from pursuing what you want. Learning to handle the challenges that come your way has a lot in common with gardening. Once you plant the seed, the process takes time, patience, and nurturing. The more significant the change, the more patience you will need before seeing tangible results. As the saying goes, "You don't pull up the radishes to see if the roots are growing."

All progress begins with a single step. No matter how small that step is, it still moves you towards your goal. That's why it is so important to focus on the present. Worry about tomorrow when it gets here — tomorrow. You cannot be alive in any moment other than the one you are in right now.

Working toward the Centre: Growth

RECOVERING A SENSE OF MEANING

CHAPTER FOURTEEN

Growth through Adversity

"Now I can look back on the positives that have emerged from the cancer, but if you'd asked me to do that while I was in treatment or even three months ago, I would have struggled with it. I was angry at cancer for disrupting my life. It's only in hindsight that I can see the gains that have come from it."

— Jennifer, 41 years old, breast cancer, 9-month survivor

"I had to extract some meaning from all that happened to me, some benefit from adversity. Looking back, I found our family became much closer as a result of the cancer. Once I realized that, I was able to move forward and find joy in my life."

— Adam, 51 years old, lymphoma, 3-year survivor

Throughout the entire recovery process, you are working to reclaim aspects of yourself. During the Inquiry Phase you're regaining your sense of self, and in the Discovery Phase you're recovering your sense of control. During these first two phases, you have the opportunity to review your current life and evaluate what you truly need and want. The Inquiry and Discovery Phases allow you to consider your pre-cancer self and compare it to the person you have become, as well as to plan ways to adapt or eliminate old patterns and outdated behaviour.

Once you enter the Growth Phase, you are halfway through your journey of transition. You have been working towards the center of the puzzle by formulating a Healing Plan and visualizing the life you want to lead. The pieces have begun falling into place, and gradually the picture of your life is taking shape. During the Growth Phase, you seek to recover a sense of meaning.

Why have we waited so long to talk in detail about something so important? Because in the early days after treatment ends, most survivors are not ready to take this step. It is simply too soon. You need the benefit of hindsight in order to digest what has happened to you, and certain things don't make sense until you have had time to absorb them. It's not until you've completed the first two phases of recovery that your spirit will be open to the call for meaning and the insights it brings. Extracting meaning from cancer takes time, but it is essential to moving forward.

"During treatment it was a matter of day-to-day survival. The processing of my experience happened afterwards. It was the biggest opportunity of my life to look back at the whole experience and see myself anew, what lessons I've learned about myself and what is important to me now."
— Gordon, 43 years old, melanoma, 2-year survivor

Our lives are in constant flux, and we have an extraordinary capacity for change. Out of chaos and confusion can come clarity, wisdom, and even the desire for greater change. But change is not synonymous with growth. There is wisdom in the adage, "Change is a given, growth is optional." We must take charge of our growth in order for our experiences to have lasting value. Finding meaning in cancer depends upon our assuming this responsibility.

This section of our book is shorter than the previous ones, but don't be deceived: shorter doesn't mean easier. After cancer, meaning may be the hardest of all things to recover, because the illness can seem so random and therefore so meaningless. Using our puzzle metaphor, meaning can remain the missing piece for years. The only way to find it is to look for it. Rarely is meaning the piece sitting in plain view on the coffee table. It may be the one that slipped under the couch or got vacuumed up by accident.

TAKING CHARGE OF GROWTH

There are two ways to view cancer, and each brings its own manner of looking at the world. Each also carries with it the possibility for living your life differently. You can choose to view cancer from the perspective that life offers continual lessons, which are opportunities for growth, or you can see your adversity as a random act of fate. On the face of it, the latter choice seems to deny meaning, but it too holds great potential for change.

MAKING MEANING

Austrian psychiatrist and author Viktor Frankl believed that human beings are fundamentally driven by their will to find meaning and purpose in life: "The way in which a man accepts his fate and all the suffering it entails, the way in which he takes up his cross, gives him ample opportunity — even under the most difficult circumstances — to add a deeper meaning to life." (1) He was a Holocaust survivor, and his personal account, *Man's Search for Meaning*, is a powerful testimony to the healing power of finding meaning in one's suffering.

Our ability to overcome a crisis in life often depends upon our capacity to make sense of it. This involves seeing beyond the present circumstances to a bigger picture in order to find or restore faith in both ourselves and a higher power. Creating meaning from challenges is a distinctly human need, and one that must be met in order for us to continue on our journey.

> *"I accepted that my cancer experience was put in my life for a bigger purpose than just to make me sick. I dove deep to try and understand what I could take away from this experience. I needed to find meaning in the pain and terror, or it all seemed so senseless."*
> — Donald, 64 years old, lung cancer, 1-year survivor

Writer and philosopher Aldous Huxley once said that experience is not what happens to you, it's what you do with what happens to you. (2) Meaning-making is not about seeing different things; rather, it involves seeing things differently. It is through finding meaning in our experiences that we learn, grow and gain a deeper understanding of our lives.

You can greatly enhance this process of growth by reframing your illness in order to look at it with new and gentle eyes. Survivors who realize they were previously travelling through life without being fully alive begin to see and live their lives differently.

> *"My outlook on life has changed since facing cancer and death. I don't rush the way I used to. I notice the intensity of colour in a flower, how clouds move in the sky, how the leaves flutter in the wind. I feel the softness of the sheets when I lie down at night. I smell the coffee for a few seconds longer as I walk past the coffee house. Life is vibrant and intense."*
>
> — Tatiana, 47 years old, breast cancer, 6-month survivor

THE VALUE OF ADVERSITY

No one welcomes adversity, but it is important to recognize adversity's role as a catalyst for significant inner growth and change.

Seeking meaning from your cancer experience may lead you to uncover strengths you didn't know you had. It may show you opportunities you didn't realize you were missing, or shift your way of thinking so that you approach your life with joy and gratitude. Pain can lead you to understand yourself better. You can transform the paralysis of fear into energy and action. None of this means that the suffering doesn't suck; it just means it has its uses. Lance Armstrong writes "I wouldn't have learned all I did if I hadn't had to contend with the cancer. I couldn't have won even one Tour without my fight, because of what it taught me ... I had a deep sense of illness, and not only wasn't I ashamed of it, I valued it above everything ... Cancer forced me to develop a plan for living ... It also taught me how to cope with losing. It taught me that sometimes the experience of losing things ... has its own value in the scheme of life." (3) We live in a world of traumas and triumphs. There are many changes that happen during the course of our lives, changes over which we have little or no control. If we can learn to explore, without judgement, the possibility that these changes have nourishing meanings and connections, then we develop resilience despite our difficulties. Resilience and an ability to adapt are necessary if we are to rise above adversity. Our efforts to find meaning are a natural and essential part of moving from coping to adapting. For survivors, recovering a sense of meaning is a crucial part of coming to terms with the changes cancer brings.

WAKING UP

Daily life is a busy undertaking, and we often sleepwalk through even the most important parts. We go to school, find a job, get married, have children, get divorced, all the while obediently following some cultural or familial script about what our lives should be like. It is possible to lose ourselves in trivia, to drown in detail, so that we have no time to stand back and appreciate the bigger picture.

Cancer shuts off the treadmill. That can be unpleasant. The treadmill was what kept you going, and everyone knows it's important to keep going. But it is only once you stop that you realize maybe walking outdoors and actually having a destination would be more exciting than running on that wretched machine every day. Cancer can be the door that leads out, causing you to turn your full attention to the present. Suddenly you see how often you have fallen into decisions rather than actively making choices. Cancer can help you decide to live each day with intention rather than running heedlessly through your life.

> *"You realize how fragile your life is. While I had known in theory to live every day to my utmost, it's not until after you've had something like this happen that you really get it. I realized that this was the life of my choosing and that I had better start enjoying it — no, really treasuring it — my kids, husband, friends, my garden, my work, whatever I do. You just don't know when it will all end."*
>
> — Sari, 49 years old, colon cancer, 4-year survivor

Cancer survivors experience real personal change. They see shifts in their attitudes, beliefs, and behaviours that would not have occurred otherwise.

They may introduce creative or spiritual elements into their lives to add richness and new meaning. They learn to turn obstacles into possibilities, limitations into strengths. Cancer can bring with it a gratitude for life, which most other people take for granted. The reality is, we are all living on borrowed time. Those who have confronted serious illness embrace their days, knowing them to be precious.

A diagnosis of cancer brings with it an acute awareness of time. Survivors report feeling as if time is running out to do what needs to be done. Many want to make the most of every remaining second. Facing death can be the push to embrace life, not just live it.

> *"You can't help but look back on your life and realize, 'Oh, I have wasted so much time!' All my regrets suddenly resurfaced and I felt a desperate urgency to act."*
>
> — Andy, 44 years old, leukemia, 9-month survivor

But embracing life might also mean *learning* how to waste time. If you are someone whose previous life was scheduled down to the minute, the idea of doing whatever comes your way, with no set plans, may be sheer pleasure. Before cancer, you may have been so wrapped up in efficiency that you never allowed yourself the luxury of taking an afternoon nap, reading a book late into the night or strolling along the lakeshore. It can seem frivolous to make time for these things in a society that values productivity. For many survivors, giving themselves permission to slow down is essential to their recovery.

CATALYSTS FOR GROWTH

Your life is a mosaic of experiences. Some events stand out more boldly or take a more dramatic shape, but each experience is an essential part of your unique life story. Every one of us encounters stumbling blocks along the way. The trick is to turn these into stepping stones. No matter what the circumstances of your life, you can find opportunities in even your most negative experiences. Problems and crises can become occasions for further understanding of yourself and of others.

There are as many ways to find meaning in cancer as there are cancer survivors. However, many survivors have found the following strategies useful:

- Take stock of your life
- Seek quiet every day
- Accept mystery
- Find the positives in your experience
- Face your mortality
- Acknowledge the mountain

Take some time to consider each of these strategies, and find the ones that appeal to you. Tailor them to your own needs as you like, or use them as springboards for your own ideas. As with other aspects of recovery, you are in charge.

Take Stock of Your Life

If you have read this far in the book, you may already have begun to take stock of your life. In this phase of recovery, too, we urge you to step back for a moment and have a look around. It will make all the difference.

> *"The bottom line is, what came out of my illness turned into my new life. I don't know if I could have recognized who I was in any other way. Nothing else would have motivated me to do the things I did. I would never have taken such risks before. I would have gone on being a high paid executive sitting in my office day after day. I wouldn't have quit my job to pursue a music writing career, as I'm doing now."*
> — Sam, 53 years old, prostate cancer, 2-year survivor

Once you are open to learning about yourself, you can begin to see the silver lining in the dark cloud of cancer. Making choices guided by what matters most to you allows you to live more directly from your heart. And when you live from your heart, anything is possible. You can rise above negative beliefs that have been passed down to you. You can participate in activities that the pre-cancer you would have never considered.

"According to my friends, the post-cancer 'me' is more fun. I'm willing to take more risks and have developed a 'seize the day' attitude. Before cancer, my life was very busy; every minute was scheduled. I still set goals and have things I want to get done, but I'm more relaxed and forgiving if things don't go as planned."

— Jana, 24 years old, lymphoma, 4-year survivor

If you're unsure about whether or not cancer has created any change in your life, ask yourself these questions: What choices have you made *because of* cancer? What happened in your life as a result? Maybe your illness *has* been more than just a blip in your personal timeline. Maybe it has been the catalyst for a new beginning.

For some survivors, cancer becomes an opportunity to acknowledge their core self, to appreciate that beneath the pain and suffering lies the bigger story of their strength and resilience.

"I've had a lot of tough times in my 32 years. I've been sick, I've been betrayed, I've been robbed — you name it — but I always knew I'd make it, I'd be okay. There is a movie called 'The Right Stuff' about what makes a good pilot. Well, I'm not a pilot, but I know that deep within my core, I have the right stuff."

— Anthony, 32 years old, lymphoma, 2-year survivor

The transition after treatment is marked by change and loss, by fear and confusion and other strong feelings. Yet many survivors speak of growth-filled, even passionate experiences that came into their lives because of cancer.

Hurtling through the Void can be terrifying, but it can also be enlightening. For all the sadness cancer brings, on the other side of loss lie insights and new perspectives on life.

"I learned how to stand up for myself, to say no when I needed to, to jump at chances when they presented themselves, and to say yes to my desires."

— Daniel, 27 years old, testicular cancer, 2-year survivor

Seek Quiet Every Day

It was St. Augustine who said, "The love of truth doth ask a holy quiet." (4) Deep self-understanding can come through regular periods of silence and introspection.

We live, for the most part, in a world full of loud distractions. The invention of the cell phone, the Blackberry and other paraphernalia has meant that we can carry our work and noise around with us everywhere. While this may be heralded as a great advance for technology, it can be soul-deadening to surround yourself with such constant interruption.

Often you don't even realize the noise around you until you begin to seek silence. Silence is like a deep breath. It refreshes the senses, calms the mind, and allows you to hear the inner voice that so wants to communicate with you. You need space to listen, and you need quiet. It is here that insights will be revealed. Whether you meditate, pray, contemplate sacred works, or just sit and enjoy the silence, you will come to appreciate this oasis of peace in your busy day.

> *"I don't try to rationalize or normalize what happened to me, but I've spent a lot of time on my own thinking about it all. I've lived through stuff I never thought I was capable of, and I've found a strength deep within me I could never have predicted."*
>
> — Lars, 49 years old, head/neck cancer, 1-year survivor

Accept Mystery

As survivors awaken to life's harsh truth of impermanence, they speak of living in mystery. They come to see the extraordinary in the ordinary, the grandeur in the commonplace. They see themselves surrounded by simple things that they suddenly recognize as amazing, even miraculous.

The reality is that we do not understand everything in our universe and probably never will. There are mysteries in life — lots of them. There are many things that scientists cannot explain. There are questions that do not have answers. This doesn't mean it is futile to ask such questions — indeed, it is in the asking itself that meaning lies. The important point to remember about mystery is that there is nothing wrong with being confused. Your confusion might be what impels you to seek answers. But once you reach the limits of understanding and realize you cannot go any further, perhaps the answer will be that life is mysterious, and that mystery is part of its beauty.

Find the Positives in Your Experience

Some survivors are adamant that they do not want to leave the experience of cancer without assigning it a positive value. Many speak of a yearning to see their suffering as having some purpose, whether that be a greater appreciation for life or the discovery of new wisdom or strength.

> *"I want to get everything I can out of this experience in terms of aware-*
> *ness, insight, or understanding. I want to leave this process feeling as if I've*
> *grown from what just happened. Otherwise, what was it all about?"*
> — Salina, 47 years old, cervical cancer, 5-month survivor

In order to find value in the experience of cancer, you might need to change the questions that you ask yourself. We turn once again to the expertise of Viktor Frankl, who practiced logotherapy, a form of psychotherapy centred on exploring meaning. Frankl believed that you would be confounded if you asked the question *What do I expect from life?* because the question itself is backwards. What you should ask instead is, *What does life expect from me?* Only then will you begin to make progress in your answers. (5)

Asking what life expects from you forces you to take responsibility for your own existence. It presumes, first and foremost, that you are here to learn from life. Life sets us tasks. It presents us with problems. It is up to us to fulfill the tasks and solve the problems. The search for meaning is what's important. The meaning you find will be specific to *your* life, not to anyone else's.

> *"There must be a purpose to the suffering that cancer brings. It's meant to*
> *make us question who we are, where we are going and who we want along*
> *for the ride. It's meant to make us better people and to improve our lives*
> *in whatever time we have left."*
> — Calen, 52 years old, melanoma, 3-month survivor

Face Your Mortality

Cancer forces you to contemplate your own mortality. However much you may try to shy away from it, death remains right there, demanding that you look it in the eye.

Death is the greatest teacher in life, but it is also the most challenging. We are terrified of dying, and we spend much of our lives trying to deny the power death holds over us. But death is also a great trickster: the more you avoid thinking about it, the less able you are to fully live your life. The author Carlos Castaneda wrote that we should carry death upon our left shoulder, struggle with it, befriend it and let it guide us through life. (6) To live in constant awareness that your existence is limited is the best way to appreciate what you have and make the best use of your time.

Their brush with death gives many cancer survivors a greater capacity to embrace and accept all of life, the joy and the sorrow, the fullness and the emptiness, the beauty and the terror. They emerge with a new level of awareness that is rich with insights and with a broader acceptance of life's daily lessons. Death can change your life if you become responsive to it. This awareness shows you that you have not lived as you might have. None of us knows when we will die, and most of us don't even believe we're going to. But when you start thinking about death, really thinking about it, you realize you must make changes now, do what you want to do. Appreciate everything. Choose happiness.

Acknowledge the Mountain

For anyone who has faced a considerable obstacle, mountain climbing is an apt metaphor for tackling difficulties. When you are diagnosed with cancer, it is as if fate plunks an enormous mountain down on your life and says *Here, climb this.* You are not given a choice. You climb.

It is only with the hindsight of recovery that you can look down and see the height of the mountain you have scaled by surviving cancer. You've made it to the top of this one. The view is breathtaking. You would never have believed you could do this. We are all far more capable and resilient than we realize, but usually we have to be forced by circumstances to find that out.

Some survivors find meaning as they acknowledge how much they have accomplished by surviving cancer. This leads to a realization: you are stronger than you thought. If you can do this, who's to say what else you can do? The next mountain you face might look less like an obstacle than a challenge.

DEALING WITH MEANINGLESSNESS

Facing death can lead you to another road, too: the belief that because we are going to die, life is meaningless. There are survivors who, try as they might, cannot find meaning in their illness. This is the second way to view cancer, not as an opportunity for growth but as a random twist of fate.

> *"I didn't spend long thinking, 'Why me?' It was a roll of the dice, just something that happened. It's not fair, but eventually, you move on into, 'Okay, now what are you going to do?' The ball has been placed in your court, and you have an opportunity to play it the way you like."*
>
> — Liane, 38 years old, leukemia, 3-year survivor

Others put the experience into context by realizing that if life is indeed random and can end at any moment, it is only sensible to appreciate every moment you have. They make meaning out of the meaningless by learning to live in the present and opening themselves to every aspect of life. Psychiatrist Dr. M. Scott Peck puts it this way: "As you struggle with the mystery of your death, you will discover the meaning of your life." (7)

The problem is that many people do not want to engage in such a struggle. Once embarked upon the road of meaninglessness, they stumble into the traps of anger, bitterness, or self-pity, which are serious impediments to growth. These attitudes are common to most survivors at one time or another along the path to recovery, but if they are held for too long they can prove challenging to even the most dedicated seekers of meaning.

Anger and Bitterness

These feelings are a reaction to the absolute injustice of cancer. Good people get cancer; healthy people who've never smoked a cigarette are diagnosed with lung cancer; people who keep a meticulously positive attitude die from the disease. Cancer is not fair. It strikes children, young parents, people who've finally reached retirement and are about to take the vacation of a lifetime.

All survivors go through a period of anger and bitterness towards the disease. It is normal and healthy to feel this way. But what will not serve you well is to get stuck here and never see the other side of your loss. It is a slippery slope from self-righteous anger to seeing yourself as a victim. Bitterness is a corrosive emotion. It will keep eating at you and trap you in the ugliness of the disease. To keep moving forward, you must come to realize that there is more to cancer than just what it takes away from you.

Self-Pity and Entitlement

The natural consequence of staying angry is to start feeling sorry for yourself. This, too, is part of the recovery process. Who has a better right to feel sorry for themselves than someone who has had cancer?

Entitlement is a form of self-pity. It is the rationale that because you have suffered, life owes you an easy time from now on. Taken to the extreme, this attitude leads some to use their cancer as an excuse. They may postpone resuming active participation in their lives, avoiding or handing off normal adult responsibilities or manipulating others, through guilt, to make few demands on them.

> *"I know I blame things that don't go my way on the cancer. If I get a bad mark on my exam I blame the cancer; if I don't have a date I blame the cancer; if I can't travel with my friends I blame the cancer. It can be an easy place to stay in. Eventually I came to understand it wasn't the cancer, it was me not accepting change."*
> — Marietta, 24 years old, lymphoma, 1-year survivor

But after a while, self-pity gets tiresome. Whining and wailing about your lot in life does nothing to improve it; it only ensures that you will remain where you are. And remaining where you are ensures that you will be unable to reframe the cancer experience and move forward. If you are bound and determined not to gain any insights from your illness, you won't. If you are certain there is nothing positive about cancer, there won't be. Only when you open your mind and heart to the possibility you might not have suffered in vain will you discover that suffering and growth walk hand in hand down the path of recovery.

LIFE'S LARGER MEANING

All transitions contain the opportunity for learning. But the possibilities are often hidden deep within the challenges. When faced with significant change, you can lose sight of life's larger meaning. Recovering a sense of meaning can put you on an active search for the gains hidden within the losses. It will take time, but the rewards are numerous. When we face hardships, we always have a choice: either we can be transformed by the experience, or we can scramble back to the familiar and let the moment pass. What will you choose?

CHAPTER FIFTEEN

From Wounds to Wisdom

"Facing my own death rocked me to my core. The one thing I got out of it is how desperate I am to really live."

   — Phillipe, 54 years old, bladder cancer, 2-month survivor

"I can't say that having cancer was a gift; it wasn't. But it did bring a number of positive things into my life. I grab life and live every day with gratitude. Cancer restored my connection with the important things in my life: my faith, my family, and my friends. It may sound crazy, but I almost feel I have an edge over others who haven't had to experience a life-threatening illness."

   — Michael, 42 years old, lymphoma, 6-month survivor

An essential component in recovering a sense of meaning is finding a door to the opportunities inherent in your cancer experience. Many insights can arise from the confusion and disorder that mark the aftermath of a life-threatening illness. Now is the time to harvest those insights.

Opening to the possibilities contained in any change is no small task. Most of us are dragged kicking and screaming to every one of life's lessons. Finding the positive in your cancer experience will take persistence. No one claims that such awareness comes easily. We acknowledge the devastation that cancer can leave in its wake. Yet we have been privileged to witness firsthand, through hundreds of survivors' testimonies, the power of the indomitable human spirit. Again and again, we've seen survivors face their limitations but choose to build on their capabilities. When the time is right, you *can* choose to extract wisdom from your wounds and strengths from your limitations. Many survivors take this step.

THE OTHER SIDE OF LOSS

The Chinese character for crisis is made up of two symbols: danger and hidden opportunity. We tend to think of illness as something uniformly negative. When we search for meaning, however, we are seeking the opportunity that lies hidden beneath the scars and side effects. We want to find a way to transform suffering into strength and beauty. In short, we are searching for hope.

Finding the insights hidden within loss can be compared to panning for gold. First you swirl the muddy water around in the pan. Once the sand settles and the water clears, you dump out the sand and water, hoping to see gold nuggets sitting in the bottom.

You'll encounter a mixture of emotions as you discover your ability to hold both sadness and wisdom within yourself, both fear and growth, both loss and new possibilities. Loss can break your heart open. Yet through that process you may discover a greater capacity for love, happiness or joy.

> "When I look back and think about how my body has changed, that I had to leave my job and how much time I've lost, I am very sad. But the other side is that I've been given all of these incredible gifts: I am exploring my writing, I am travelling more, and I've just begun a relationship with a very caring person."
>
> — Janet, 38 years old, lymphoma, 4-year survivor

Some survivors are adamant that there are *no* gifts in cancer, in having to endure that much suffering and pain. Others use the term freely and truly feel cancer was a blessing.

> "I know some people hate it when they hear me say, 'Cancer was a real gift in my life,' but it was. It changed everything. Not only is my lifestyle

healthier now, but so is my family's. Our attitude toward life is to keep liv-
ing fully each day."

— Marcyn, 41 years old, ovarian cancer, 6-year survivor

Other survivors cite gains such as strengthened relationships, a greater commitment to their work, deeper compassion, better health, more enjoyment
of physical activity, a more profound understanding of spirituality, and a new
ability to appreciate the moment. But it takes time and effort to see these
gains and to acknowledge cancer's hand in them.

LEARNING LINKS THE OLD AND THE NEW

Many academic theories exist about how we learn. There are also popular
and cultural beliefs about the role life's lessons play in our growth and development. Some people believe that the lessons we need will present themselves in various forms until we have finally attended to them. Others believe
that our lives are defined by the challenges we face.

In her book *Choices,* author Melody Beattie acknowledges, "Every step
of the way there is something to learn. But just when you think you've got
them all under your belt, another lesson comes your way. I kept waiting for
the lessons to stop, and I would get moments of rest, play and respite. Until
the winds blew another lesson my way." (1)

Change can stimulate learning, and learning can in turn initiate
greater change. One of the paradoxes of learning is that sometimes we
are required to unlearn a belief or attitude to make room for something
new. By giving up some components of your old self, you allow a new
self to form.

"I learned to be more compassionate and gentler with myself. I learned
to trust that I was wise and knew what I needed in my life better than
anyone else. I learned that I could ask for and accept help, and people
would still love me. I learned I had more love in my life than I had ever
realized. I learned that I could survive periods of despair and come out
the other side and carry on. I learned it's impossible to skip and not

*smile at the same time (try it, you'll see!). I am stronger than I ever knew
I could be. I am more courageous than I realized."*
> — Mary, 48 years old, breast cancer, 7-year survivor

As you open to change, you will develop a new level of trust in yourself and
in your abilities to handle physical and emotional challenges. Your new sense
of self can assist you to see the future as an adventure. Some survivors feel
freer in themselves; they are willing to take more liberties and to act on a
leap of faith.

*"I'm not a completely different person, but I am a better person. My life is
definitely not what it was. It's enhanced."*
> — Mathew, 45 years old, head/neck cancer, 6-month survivor

As with every stage of the recovery process, seeking meaning in your experience may also stimulate fears.

*"When I took the time to really think about everything that happened to
me and what I had learned from it, the last thing I expected was to see how
afraid I was. I suppose fear is a good teacher, but a demanding one, too.
While I was discovering how strong I was, I was also staring at all of my
vulnerabilities. It was unsettling."*
> — Shirley, 39 years old, leukemia, 4-month survivor

You will need to come armed to this battle. The best way is to identify your
fears, look at them and decide what to do with them. Facing down your fears
shows them you are strong enough to handle them. You may feel that cancer
has left you weak rather than strong. But maybe you're just not looking in
the right place for your strength.

HARVESTING YOUR STRENGTHS

While everyone's life involves a series of changes that unfold over a lifetime,
the adversities that accompany cancer may require survivors to develop

longer-range adaptive skills. Invaluable resources to assist you in developing resilience lie well within your reach. They are your strengths, and they are found within you.

"You don't know the true strength of the human body until there is a need in your life to test it."
— Robert, 48 years old, brain cancer, 1-year survivor

Out of the experience of surviving cancer can come a new level of trust in yourself. You have been tested and now have a whole new appreciation of what you can handle. Recognizing your resilience can bring both comfort and a new perspective.

"I have more confidence in my ability to deal with almost anything. I have a new trust and understanding of my body and my relationship to life. I had never looked at death before. It terrified me. Now I've faced it, studied it, and learnt from it. I have a conviction to live life with gusto like I've never had before."
— Julie, 33 years old, lymphoma, 3-month survivor

As humbling as it is to feel lost, weak and vulnerable, such wounding can be the very doorway that leads us to profound strength. This does not glorify or in any way minimize the pain and suffering that cancer brings. What it does is acknowledge the reality expressed by many survivors that they were able to take strength from their misfortune, that their lives after cancer changed for the better. In her book *The Alchemy of Illness,* Kat Duff writes, "Even at my sickest when I was spending the majority of my time in bed, I knew my illness was showing me facets of truth I had missed." (2)

What strengths might you be able to rely upon after your illness? There are many, but let's look at three commonly cited by survivors:

- Clarity
- Compassion
- Enhanced spiritual awareness

Clarity

Being thankful for what you have is not always easy after you have survived cancer. Often what you had has been changed or taken away from you, causing you to feel resentful and angry.

Here, again, is attitude, and the choice that every survivor must make: to be bitter over your loss or grateful for what you have. Gratitude is central to keeping your priorities clear and living in the moment because it requires you to be thankful for things you may otherwise have taken for granted.

> *"Theory is so different from experience. Sure, we all say how important love, family, and friends are, but it was only after I had cancer that I began to understand just how true that is. I now have a greater sense of how brief and precious life can be. It has made me so grateful for what I have. I want to appreciate and honour life in all aspects, my life in particular."*
> — Rashida, 58 years old, cervical cancer, 8-year survivor

Clarity comes from reframing your cancer experience, finding your strengths and harvesting the insight you've gained about what brings meaning and purpose to life. With the support of family and friends, many survivors use their cancer experience as an opportunity to rediscover who they are, what they want, where they are going and who they want to be there with them.

Compassion

The yearning within the human heart to reach out to others in pain is part of our capacity for empathy. Yet deep compassion can come only through your own experience. When a friend's parent dies, you are sympathetic, but you don't really grasp such loss until it happens to you. The same can be said for any profound grief or loss.

Thanks to their own struggles with cancer, many survivors discover newfound empathy and compassion for others. Indeed, they develop a new tenderness for life in general. They become more spacious in their thinking, acknowledging that the emotional storms that blow through their own lives likely gust through the lives of others, too.

"I never really knew how others with cancer felt before I got cancer. Two people at work had cancer, but I didn't know what to say or do. I feel sad that I wasn't there for them, now that I realize how much they could have used the extra support."

— Brandy, 38 years old, breast cancer, 1-year survivor

Spiritual teachings acknowledge the role of suffering in spiritual growth. Suffering and compassion work together. Suffering forces us to experience our own vulnerability, and through that we come to understand the vulnerability of others. It takes great courage to open up to suffering, both your own and that of others. Fear holds us back and keeps us silent, but compassion enables us to step into the world and face uncertainty.

"I realized I could love and be loved. I opened my heart and began to reach out to others with a new understanding of illness, pain, sadness, fear, and an intense joy for living each day. When you've been there, you can't help but feel compassion for others who are travelling the same road."

— Charlene, 49 years old, leukemia, 4-year survivor

Compassion recognizes that we all strive to do the best we can within the limits of our current beliefs and capabilities. Compassion for yourself and your own vulnerabilities can be a great spiritual resource during this time of transition. The more loving-kindness you can give to yourself, the more able you are to extend it to others. In her book *When Things Fall Apart*, Pema Chödrön teaches us that the noble heart is one that sheds its armour, opening itself fearlessly to both heartache and delight. She encourages us to embrace the pain of our experience: "Instead of fending it off and hiding from it, we could open our hearts and allow ourselves to feel that pain, feel it as something that will soften and purify us and make us far more loving and kind." (3)

Compassion does not mean letting people walk all over you or putting up with destructive behaviour. It means making room in your heart for kindness and understanding. The poet Rumi wrote, "Out beyond ideas of wrongdoing and rightdoing, there is a field. I'll meet you there. When the soul lies down in that grass, the world is too full to talk about." (4) Rumi understood that judgments — those we make about others and ourselves — harm our spirit. Be gentle and patient with yourself. Create an open attitude by deciding to learn from your mistakes and move on rather than judging yourself.

> *"I think I'm a better person since cancer. I understand suffering at a very visceral level now. Before, I used to race by people and not pay much attention to them. Now I slow down and I notice who walks with a limp, who needs a little extra time to cross the street, and who looks like they may be hurting inside."*
> — Maureen, 49 years old, brain cancer, 2-year survivor

Compassion motivates many survivors into volunteer and advocacy work with other cancer patients. Many express a desire to help ease the recovery transition for others.

> *"Having faced dying at 43, I suddenly began to appreciate life and to see more clearly than before that life is about love and compassion, not about acquiring and winning. Whenever possible, I reach out to others, and I never try to go back on a generous impulse."*
> — Peggy, 46 years old, breast cancer, 3-year survivor

Showing compassion will take you farther along the path of connection to all aspects of yourself and ultimately result in a feeling of greater wholeness. By moving out from beneath your own shadow to a place of generosity, you will be overcoming self-imposed boundaries and limitations as well as the limits imposed on you by others. Indeed you are creating new possibilities and then achieving them.

Enhanced Spiritual Awareness

Many cancer survivors experience a renewed or enhanced spiritual awareness. Turning to God or spiritual practices for comfort and solace can help you cope with the changes cancer brings. Some survivors speak of having an epiphany or a mystical vision that brought them to a new level of spiritual awakening. Others discover a deeper sense of meaning and purpose to their lives.

A sense of spiritual well-being can give you immense hope for tomorrow. Exploring, acknowledging or reclaiming your spiritual awareness can be a source of strength not only during recovery but for the rest of your life.

FOOD FOR THOUGHT

Perhaps you have never thought about cancer in positive terms. Words like gift, gain, insight, and strength may have never matched up with this disease in your mind. Now is the time to try out these ideas and see how they work for you.

Here are some questions to get you started. Take time to ponder them, and record your thoughts in your recovery journal.

- What have you gained from your cancer experience?
- How have you become stronger because of cancer?
- Did cancer reveal strengths you never realized you had?
- What kind of learning has come from your cancer experience? Can you relate any insights that you've had specifically to your cancer experience?
- Do you have compassion for yourself and your current limitations?
- Has cancer influenced your compassion for others?

The insights we glean from the events that occur in our lives help us to move beyond obstacles. They make it possible for us to discover who we were, who we've become and where we're going. Whether you harvest significant insights from your cancer experience or simply take time to appreciate each day, recovering a sense of meaning is an essential aspect of healing. From meaning comes purpose, which allows you to make life changes you may only have dreamed of before. Finding meaning gives you a reason to grow and to change.

Attentive Walking

As you take your daily walk, give yourself permission to change direction, explore new surroundings, or make a detour. Every small change of habit creates the possibility for larger changes. If you've ever walked a straight path, you will know that it can get monotonous. It's the twists and turns that keep things interesting, and often the greatest surprises come when you get off the well-worn path. *Just keep walking.*

The Five-Question Check-In

As you complete your five-question check-in, notice which answers reveal hidden strengths or positive changes in your life. Become conscious of which questions inspire you to explore aspects of yourself you hadn't been aware of before. You may come up with insights that you would never have expected.

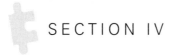

SECTION IV

Seeing the Whole Picture: Reflection

RECOVERING A SENSE OF THE FUTURE

CHAPTER SIXTEEN

Living with Uncertainty

"It's the uncertainty that's hard to deal with. My faith in the future was shattered overnight, and I'm not sure what direction to move in next. I find I'm holding my breath waiting for something terrible to happen."

— Alfred, 36 years old, lymphoma, 9-week survivor

"I can honestly say I don't worry about my future. I know there are no guarantees; the cancer could come back, but then again maybe it won't. I'm living my life, and I don't worry about things I can't control. There's freedom in that attitude."

— Faith, 51 years old, melanoma, 3-year survivor

We come now to the final phase of the recovery process, the Reflection Phase. In this chapter we will be considering the future, that elusive place many cancer survivors dread thinking about. Part of this phase involves reflecting on where you've been and what might come next for you. Part of it involves learning how to handle uncertainty. Paradoxically, to recover a sense of the future you must learn how to live in the present moment. The ultimate goal of the Reflection phase is a sense of inner peace. Can inner peace and uncertainty co-exist? Absolutely.

No one knows what will happen tomorrow or how much time any of us actually has left. Most of us do our best to ignore this. Cancer survivors don't have that luxury. Worrying about the future won't do much good; your anxiety will only interfere with your enjoyment of the present. Yet if you never think about the future, you can neither set goals nor have a vision for your life.

During treatment, most survivors simply live from one day to the next. But part of recovery — of resuming everyday life — necessarily involves looking ahead. How far ahead you want to look is up to you. The future can encompass tomorrow or next week, or it can reach into the distance. Whether you plan for next weekend, next week or the next five years, the key in this phase is to regain the sense that you have a future — one that you will have a hand in shaping.

> *"I struggled with my belief in the future for quite a while. But I started planning my weekends, then my next holiday, and eventually my vision of a fulfilling life. I actually find the thought of having limited time brings very clear focus to life plans and decisions."*
>
> — Jeremy, 51 years old, lung cancer, 2-year survivor

FEAR OF THE FUTURE

For many survivors, the whole idea of the future is fraught with fears of recurrence and impending death. They refuse to think past the present moment. They struggle to maintain their world as it was. While learning to live one day at a time is an important technique for finding pleasure in life, this is not what these survivors experience. They attempt to eliminate uncertainty by becoming inflexible about the natural fluctuations in life and try to strong-arm their cancer into submission.

The problem is, this approach doesn't work — or at least, not for long. You can't move forward if you are constantly looking over your shoulder. The only voice you will hear in your head is the voice of fear, telling you that planning for the future is futile. And that is no help at all.

Another common reaction is for survivors to cling to their pre-cancer life, which is now viewed through distinctly rose-tinted lenses. They wish everything could go back to the way it used to be. They long for the innocence and security they see as coming from not having to face your own mortality — even if that innocence and security are false. But this nostalgia, the yearning to turn back the clock, brings unnecessary pain and suffering. As much as you want life to return to the way it was, wishing will not make it so. Attaching yourself to your life before cancer will lead to more fear, more resistance and more avoidance of the changes that have occurred.

WHEN PLANNING MEETS ANXIETY

None of us can escape the fact that contemporary North American society is future-oriented. We buy on credit, plan our vacations, set goals and save for our retirement. There is very little we can do without first planning ahead.

Once your cancer treatments are finished, it is not unusual for family and friends to want to start making future plans that include you. For them, such planning is partly an act of hope and partly a desire to put cancer firmly in the past. They assume you are eager to do the same. They may have no idea of your anxiety about the future or your loss of faith in its existence.

When planning by your family or your partner clashes with your vulnerability, the result can be conflict and, over the longer term, relationship problems. While your partner rests easy in the notion that the cancer is now over, you have no such certainty. For example, Kenny and his wife were both close to finishing their university degrees and had offers of good starting positions with a major company. But he was unwilling to consider returning to university to finish his last year.

> *"What if it's all for nothing. I finish school, I get a job and the cancer recurs. Maybe I don't have much time left. I'm going to quit school, go travelling and enjoy my life."*
> — Kenny, 24 yeas old, lymphoma, 6-month survivor

It's crucial to take the time you need to recover, and if such clashes continue you may need to seek professional help. However, some survivors find it is a partner, family member or friend who finally helps them change their attitude.

*"I was told by my dad, 'Son, you can feel sad for a while, kick, cry, scream if you
want to, but at some point you have to begin pulling your life back together.'"*
— Peter, 36 years old, testicular cancer, 8-month survivor

If you intend to resume your role in your family and/or your workplace,
you will need at some point to transform your fear of the future into energy
that motivates you forward. It is healthy to plan for the future. It is an act of
faith in your life.

*"I need plans; they give me direction and provide order in my life. They fuel
the hope I need to believe I really do have a future."*
— Rebecca, 48 years old, ovarian cancer, 2-month survivor

FACING THE FUTURE WITH CURIOSITY AND HOPE

Whether you see yourself as a warrior or a peacekeeper, you must develop the
skills to face the future fearlessly. But fearlessness can only be cultivated from
within. Facing your fear doesn't mean that it will diminish. What *will* change is
your response to it. When fear bares its face, try to meet it with curiosity and
tenderness. Observe how and when it comes, and when it leaves. Fear causes
other possibilities to shrink; you pull back instead of opening up. Because fear
creates insecurity and anxiety, it can narrow your view of the future. None of
us can depend for our security on the external world or on other people.
Security comes from developing a solid, peaceful courage within.

Fearlessness means facing uncertainty with optimism. It means taking that
first step, even though you're afraid, and moving forward with confidence. It
means meeting whatever challenge presents itself with courage and fortitude.
You must be brave to hold onto the life you want to live. Fearlessness means
finding hope in the future even though you're unsure of what that future holds.

*"My warrior spirit tends to come forth during times of fear in my life. I
decided to let it fill me up so that I could tackle the problems ahead. Living
life fearlessly is my way of diving head first into the future."*
— Olivia, 49 years old, breast cancer, 4-year survivor

Fear is an emotion, and like all emotions, it will come and go. When you sit back and observe your feelings, you will see how you can vacillate between joy one moment and intense fear the next. It is when you become too attached to an emotion — any emotion — that you create pain for yourself. Wanting life to be filled only with happy moments is unrealistic too. And when we try to suppress fear or sadness, these emotions are bound to reappear.

The truth is that we are all afraid sometimes. But fearlessness is not an impossible ideal. It is an attitude that can be cultivated by learning a few strategies for facing down your fears.

> *"There is a whole attitude factor to consider. Optimism, hope, the will to live, courage, faith in oneself, and the belief that life is beautiful and worthwhile; these are the attitudes that propel me into the future."*
> — Jason, 41 years old, colon cancer, 3-month survivor

In every situation, we have a choice: to be afraid of the future or to hope for the best. To choose hope is to take a step towards healing.

CULTIVATING FEARLESSNESS

It is possible to face all of what life throws at you, including illness, dying and death, with courage. There are many strategies available to you. Here we will consider some of the strategies survivors have found most useful.

Before you read any further, we suggest that you review our suggestions for dealing with fear from Chapter 9. In that chapter we discussed the fear of recurrence survivors encounter in the earlier phases of recovery. This fear changes as recovery progresses, and thus needs to be addressed in different ways. However, many of the tools we outlined in Chapter 9 are equally applicable in the Reflection Phase of recovery. These include relaxation, movement, creativity, faith, facing your fear, letting go, having a touchstone, and using affirmations.

Take charge of your health. Taking action on your Healing Plan and Vision Statement will keep your health at the forefront of your life and motivate you to regularly re-examine your priorities. When you take charge of your health, you regain a sense of trust in yourself and in your ability to face the unknown future.

Know what sustains you. Where do you go when you need support? What gives you hope? Perhaps it is your faith in God; your trust in yourself, modern medicine, or your support team; or a combination of all of these things. Ask yourself what sustains you: that is the place you must go when you are afraid.

Focus on hope. Psychologists tell us that what we focus on increases. If you focus all of your energy on fear, your fear will escalate. So why not focus on hope? Hope is a vital ingredient in creating a vision of a new normal and of a future that is as good as, or better than, the past. Considering the future possibilities available to you enables you to make choices and perhaps even to nudge some events into being.

> *"Despite a recurrence of breast cancer, I still believe I have a long future ahead of me. I keep doing the things I love. I set new goals every New Year's eve and try to achieve them. They keep me focusing forward instead of fearful about my past."*
>
> — Caroline, 50 years old, breast cancer, 4-year survivor

Make a place for your fear. Some survivors confine the time and space in which they allow themselves to feel fear. This way, they know that fear will not take over their lives. One survivor told us that when she started obsessing about the cancer, she would go to a corner of her garden where she allowed herself to cry and to think about her fears. She allowed this there and only there. Once she left that spot, she would symbolically leave her fear behind and get on with her life.

Speak to your fear. You may find it helpful to develop a saying, affirmation, prayer, or mantra to use each time your fear arises. A strong and powerful statement such as *I'm moving forward* can keep hope front and center. Often a quick *Stop!* will halt the escalating fear and bring you back to the moment.

Use compassion, your greatest survivor strength. Develop a compassionate attitude toward your fear. Fear is the natural reaction to an uncertain future. When you befriend your fear and soften towards it instead of resisting it, you come to realize that there is room in life for everything: for fear, grief, joy, and delight. The more you can open yourself to your fear, the more manageable it will become.

> *"The elusive and deadly nature of cancer can be terrifying. I didn't want to live in constant fear of a recurrence. I refused to let it get the best of me and control the rest of my life; it had taken enough already. I choose to live each day in joy and tenderness for myself and others, not in terror."*
> — Daphne, 58 years old, colon cancer, 9-month survivor

Trust in yourself and in your ability to handle what comes your way. Many survivors pray for courage and for grace: the courage to handle each trial and to never give up; grace in each moment.

Let time help you. Fear does diminish with time. The passage of time pulls us forward and reminds us that there is life beyond cancer. Time allows the flow of everyday circumstances to re-enter our lives. Life moves on, and so must we.

Of course, you may experience moments of backsliding into fear. Some days you'll feel steady on your feet. On others you may feel as if your shoelaces are tied together. The adage "This too shall pass" is particularly helpful when it comes to facing your fear.

> *"I couldn't continue to fight the fear. I was exhausted, and I was shrinking from life. I had to redefine what I thought cancer was and build a new agreement with it. I started living with it instead of being constantly opposed to it. From that moment on, life changed and my fear lessened. My fear and I live side by side."*
> — Rennie, 43 years old, colorectal cancer, 4-year survivor

LIVING WITH UNCERTAINTY

As we have said many times in this book, change is a constant in human lives. No one knows what will happen next. "We are changing," wrote the novelist D.H. Lawrence, "we have got to change, and we can no more help it than leaves can help turning yellow and coming loose in autumn." (1) For many people, the primary dilemma that accompanies change is the uncertainty it brings. But the ability to be flexible while pursuing your healing goals means being open to whatever may come.

Over and over in our lives we are surprised by the unforeseen, many times pleasantly so. More often, however, we remember the tragedies, because they brought us suffering or pain. It is only with hindsight that we are able to recognize growth in these experiences and lay them to rest. Cancer may have knocked the wind out of your sails, but now, with the breeze at your back, it is time to re-jig your commitment to living and set sail into the unknown future.

In his book *The Way of Transition*, William Bridges acknowledges the pain of uncertainty: "What was so hard was not steering [the course] — being surrounded by uncertainty, full of uncertainty, weighed down by uncertainty. Although I didn't know how I was going to manage it, I knew that dealing successfully with the transition was going to require me to accept uncertainty as my new reality." (2)

Few people have an easy time coping with the unknown. The good news is that acknowledging your discomfort with uncertainty is the first step toward coming to grips with it. Once you're there, you can begin to map out a strategy.

"Not knowing is the true condition of everything in life. None of us knows what tomorrow will bring. Accepting that helps me to deal with the uncertainty."
— Tanya, 43 years old, thyroid cancer, 6-month survivor

After cancer, the unpredictability of life is no longer an abstract concept. It's real, and it's happening to you. There are no guarantees, no guidelines, and no magic pill that can ensure a disease-free future. The challenge is to learn to live with cancer, rather than living in fear of it. Vancouver psychologist Lee Pulos states, "I tell all my patients, 'Don't breathe life into the past; understand it, move forward and create your new reality, your new outcome. Don't breathe life into what was; breathe life into the future that you want to step into.'" (3)

Worrying about the unknown eats away at your heart, your mind and your spirit, and eventually at your health. The uncertainty of tomorrow may be an uncomfortable place to live in for a while. But struggling to hold onto what you know won't work. Life has changed. So have you. Moving into what's next with curiosity and openness is difficult, but it may bring many delightful surprises. Often life has a grander plan for us than we can even imagine.

> *"I must do all I can in this day to love, and yet still be prepared for tomorrow.*
> *I plan with intention, not with expectation of an outcome I can't control."*
> — Reuben, 55 years old, prostate cancer, 2-year survivor

In Chapter Twelve, we presented a guided process for creating a picture of what living well looks like for you. We cannot stress strongly enough how a vision of what's possible can sustain you when you are afraid. If you can see the direction forward, you can move forward. Otherwise, you will continue to wander. There are three things in life that can provide you with security: knowing who you are, knowing where you are, and knowing where you're going. When you take a bold step toward life, your fear of the future will decrease and your sense of what's possible will expand.

Worries are like hungry lions, stalking us, ready to pounce. Our imaginations can run wild with frightening images: losing a job, never finding a partner, not having enough money, getting sick again, dying. In those moments of intense worry, when fear has ambushed you and contemplating the future is too terrifying, step back from it all and stop trying to figure out the whole picture. Focus on the present. Pay attention to right now. Say to yourself *At this moment, I am okay.* Take a deep breath and then exhale all of the fear and anguish of wondering what tomorrow may bring.

> *"Having gone through cancer gives me a sense of freedom. What's the point*
> *of living half a life because you're scared of something you can't control?*

Sure, I'm afraid of tomorrow, but that makes me more passionate about living fully today."

— Sin-Yu, 54 years old, ovarian cancer, 4-year survivor

All survivors live in cancer's shadow. However, a healthy acceptance of uncertainty allows you to transform your fearful "What ifs?" into the more positive and life-affirming "What next?"

"I came to the place where I could accept not knowing. It wasn't easy in the beginning, but it's where I live now. My fear is quieter. It pops up every once in a while, but I understand dying a little better, and I believe in life after death. It helps to tone down the fear."

— Josie, 48 years old, melanoma, 5-year survivor

FAITH *IN* RATHER THAN FEAR *OF*

Faith and fear can coexist. The two run on parallel tracks throughout your life: you can experience faith in yourself, in your health, in your ability to heal, and in your future despite your fears of recurrence and of the unknown. You can decide to let the faith that exists deep within you be your guide. Faith requires relinquishing control, however, and trusting that life will unfold as it should is not easy. Loosening your grip enough to walk into the unknown will take real courage.

"The fear of recurrence is not something you can just ignore. It's like the fear of walking down the street at night and worrying that somebody might jump you. The thing is, you can always choose which street you're going to walk down. Even if you know fear is there, you don't have to live according to its rules."

— Drew, 46 years old, brain cancer, 2-year survivor

PAY ATTENTION

It can take a catastrophe for us to recognize that we are often bystanders in our own lives. Awareness, consciousness, being awake, being mindful, paying attention: these terms acknowledge the importance of cultivating a heightened attentiveness to what is happening to us and around us in the present moment. When we are mindful, we observe our thoughts and feelings, not evaluating them but simply letting them move through us. We start to see things as they actually are, rather than how we wish them to be. This helps us gain perspective so that we can choose our responses.

> *"I felt as if I had been sleeping through my life. Suddenly I had cancer, and I woke up to wanting to understand my life and to participate in all it had to offer."*
> — Liane, 38 years old, leukemia, 3-year survivor

Living consciously gives you confidence that you are using your time well. Even more significantly, it allows you to connect with your authentic self. When you exist in concert with yourself and your surroundings, you become consciously aware of what contributes to your healing.

When you start to pay attention, you may realize that a lot of your time is spent regretting the past and worrying about the future. Both states take you out of the present moment. One of the core Buddhist principles reminds us that if you miss the moment, you miss your life. Life is a series of moments strung together. Recovering a sense of the future will require you to reach for the future, honour the past, but live in the now.

Your daily attentive walk and five-question check-in encourage you to pay attention to what is happening in your current reality on many levels: physical, emotional, spiritual and social. What they really ask you to do is to become more present in your life.

REFLECTION

In all of our lives, there are times for action and times for stillness. The Reflection Phase of recovery is a time for contemplation. Our achievement-oriented society makes it challenging to even find such time, but reflection is an essential part of integrating change. Every now and then, we need to stop, take a breath, and look around at what is going on. Sometimes it is not until you look back that you can see how far you have come. While you are in recovery, reflection allows you to recognize the healing that has occurred as well as the areas that still need to be addressed.

The earlier phases of our four-part recovery program focus on working, doing, and growing. Now we move into a being, resting and evaluating phase. When you reach this stage of recovery, you may be tempted to skip the reflection process, figuring you are already close enough to establishing your new normal. But reflecting on your experience, the changes you've gone through, your choices, your intentions and your actions gives you precious feedback — in fact, necessary feedback — that allows you to draw conclusions and bring closure to your experience. When you reflect consciously on the transition process, you can see clearly where you've been and where you are going.

> *"I hear all the time that you learn from your experiences, but I can experience the same thing over and over again and never learn anything until I stop and reflect. I learn from a friend when we sit and talk about what happened; then I am able to see and hear what I am really saying about it. It is through reflection that I identify insights."*
>
> — Hope, 49 years old, breast cancer, 6-year survivor

Reflection is the doorway into the deepest aspects of self-awareness. Once you have reached this phase of the recovery process, you will need to find a quiet place where you can be alone with your thoughts. Ask yourself *What did I set out to do during recovery? What did I achieve? What new insights have I gained?* Listen carefully for the answers. As you integrate them into your consciousness they will become incorporated into the new you.

FINDING INNER PEACE

If you recall our list of survivor wants from Chapter Two, inner peace was one of the ultimate wants. Inner peace is, indeed, the main goal of the Reflection Phase. Often we rush around trying to get things done in the hope that eventually we can stop, relax, and find some peace. But peace is actually a state of mind we can learn to tap into.

Peace hides beneath the noise in our heads and the constant noise of the external world. You may need to dig deep if you wish to find it. Inner peace involves a calm mind, an open heart and a feeling of being centred. Being in a serene atmosphere can help you feel peaceful. However, a sense of peace does not depend on outer circumstances. There may be times when you are surrounded by chaos but feel healthy and strong deep within. There are also times when you must take charge of your own inner peace, making a conscious effort to find serenity.

"I feel peaceful when I slow down, open up and connect with myself and the world. My thoughts can easily spiral into a state of frenzy, but I can stop them now and bring myself back to the quiet."
— Courtney, 50 years old, ovarian cancer, 18-month survivor

The feeling of being at peace is usually attained during times of deep connection, when you are at your most grounded: walking in nature, creating, praying, being in sync with your partner. Moments of gratitude can also be times of peace.

"I feel most at peace when I am dancing, connecting to the rhythm of the music and the flow of the energy in my body. During those times life is at its most glorious. I feel immense gratitude for being alive."
— Sabrina, 39 years old, cervical cancer, 3-year survivor

Can such peace exist in a life that is full of uncertainty? In *A Path with Heart*, author Jack Kornfield writes that we can find inner peace only when we embrace life's opposites: birth and death, joy and suffering, the known and the uncertain. (4) It's not until we loosen our grip on life and allow it to unfold naturally that we can relax into peacefulness.

Just as your journey through the Void of transition takes time and requires you to complete several steps, accepting cancer is a gradual movement from struggle and suffering to simply living with what is. With acceptance, you no longer need to judge your cancer experience, assigning labels of "good" or "bad" to each scenario. Acceptance allows you to make peace with cancer.

You give the story of cancer its place. You are not the cancer, but it has been a part of your life. Stepping into this peacefulness doesn't mean that everything is suddenly fine — you still have to deal with life as it is — but you can move forward with greater confidence and less fear of the future. This is another of the many paradoxes at the centre of life: in order to take charge, you must let go.

In her book *How to Ride a Dragon*, Michelle Tocher talks of coming to terms with cancer: "Coming into the heart of the dragon is a story of acceptance. The women who struggled against the dragon of cancer ultimately went from trying to kill it to accepting it, and when they did, their hearts opened. As they greeted the dragon, they greeted themselves …What it means is that the struggle against themselves ended; the slayer and the enemy 'died' together. The women came to see that even death was not against them. It was a mysterious way of bringing them closer to themselves, closer to home. So began the cooperation that transformed the deadly dragon into a beautiful companion and the dragon slayer into a brave and gentle rider, humbled by the mystery of life." (5)

As you grow more comfortable with letting go of things that are beyond your control, you open the door to peace. The future is unknowable, but you can begin to trust it again. You can bring to it a sense of wonder, an eagerness for mystery, and even a willingness to believe in miracles.

INTEGRATION

During the Reflection Phase of recovery, survivors speak of a new level of contentment that stems from an acceptance of themselves and others. They have navigated significant physical changes, negotiated with strong emotions, faced loss and in some cases despair, and reached a positive new place from which to live. Some have learned for the first time to trust in their own authority.

In the early days of transition, many people struggle to get their old lives back. By this stage of the game, you come to realize that old concepts, ideals, habits, and emotional patterns no longer fit. The time for moving on to a new life is at hand. There may still be days when you wrestle with fear, anger or denial. But you have formed a deep commitment by now to your ongoing recovery and your dreams for a healthy life. Your commitment gives you great personal power and a sense of responsibility to yourself.

Integration is not a place you reach. Rather, it is a process of daily choices and decisions that eventually combine your pre- and post-cancer experiences into a harmonious whole. Within this harmony lies an acceptance of the irrevocable nature of the disease, the strengths and limitations that accompany survival, and the positive and negative consequences that follow in cancer's wake. You have been on an incredible adventure, and despite the fact that you did not choose to undertake this quest, it has still brought you new strengths and insights.

"There is a synthesis of the me before and after cancer. I can see the old but like the new me. I look at the process of taking the best and moving forward and admire the resiliency of the human spirit."
— Christina, 56 years old, colorectal cancer, 1-year survivor

The process of integration sometimes resembles a painting effect called pentimento. Long ago, canvases were recycled and old paintings were painted over to create a new work. But as the top layers of paint wore away or became transparent with age, the painting's owner would get a surprise: an earlier painting was revealed.

As you layer your past with new habits, ideas, beliefs and people, you may still catch fleeting glimpses of the painting beneath: your former self. This may make you nostalgic or sad. But more likely, these glimpses will confirm to you the rightness of your new painting. The brilliant colours and textures that you have chosen appeal to you. In the end, what you create becomes a true integration of the best of the old with the promise of the new.

Through reflection, you will bring together new perspectives and insights gleaned from your previous life's lessons. You will integrate what has emerged from your cancer experience and create a new wisdom for yourself. Once all the pieces of the puzzle are in place, you will be able to see the whole picture, though it will differ from the original. Who you were immediately after treatment is not who you will be one, two or many years afterwards. Healing after cancer is a journey toward regaining wholeness. But wholeness is a concept that evolves as life shifts and swirls. We are constantly changing, facing new challenges, moving through transitions and reshaping our picture. There are many possible futures. Step into the one you choose, trusting life's changes and knowing that you have the tools to handle them, the strength to move through them and an unshakeable belief in yourself.

CHAPTER SEVENTEEN

Don't Go Back to Sleep

"I promised I'd be gentler with myself, have more fun, and follow my heart more and my head less. Sometimes that gets lost in the little things of my day. It takes effort to remember, but it's worth it."

— Penelope, 32 years old, leukemia, 1-year survivor

"I'd like to think I don't make promises I can't keep. I made these promises to myself, and I swore I'd keep them as time went on, that I wouldn't forget. So I set up little foolproof ways to keep my promises. I write them in my day-timer on the first day of each month. That way I see them before me and they remind me not to forget."

— Cheri, 43 years old, cervical cancer, 2-year survivor

You have come a long way in your recovery by the time you reach the Reflection Phase. You have re-established faith in yourself and in your capacity to heal. You no longer rely only on external voices of authority, but have learned to listen to your own inner voice. You have developed faith in your Healing Plan and in your ability to get support and address obstacles. You have faith in life and are taking strong, confident steps to pursue the life you want.

Over the course of your recovery journey, you will have discovered that time is a great healer. Time mends wounds, both physical and emotional. Time mitigates fear. But time can also make you forget. Sometimes this is a blessing, but sometimes it means that all that gratitude for each moment you were certain would never leave you and all those insights you gleaned from your cancer experience slowly wane, then disappear. You go to your check-ups, each one less scary than the last. Your health returns and you begin to take it for granted. Old habits reassert themselves. The days rush past in a whirlwind of grocery shopping, work and traffic jams, and at some point you realize with dismay that the learning you amassed from the cancer experience has been buried amidst the chaos of everyday life.

> *"The old cliché about stopping and smelling the roses is so true once you face death. You promise yourself you'll slow down; life passes by too quickly. But then life does start to pass by and you move quickly with it. It takes a conscious effort to spend more time with the people you love or appreciate the small pleasures in life. It doesn't just happen."*
> — Charlene, 67 years old, breast cancer, 3-year survivor

Cancer is a fight for your life. It is intense, focused, and requires every part of you. But the fight does end, and life goes on. You regain strength during recovery and you make promises to yourself: you won't sweat the small stuff, you won't worry so much, you will wring every ounce out of the present moment. And for a while, you do.

> *"Once you face cancer you really 'get life.' You get it like never before. And you know others who have faced any kind of life-threatening illness or event get it as well. But getting it and keeping it foremost in the centre of your life is very challenging."*
> — Chad, 43 years old, colorectal cancer 4-year survivor

Your awareness of the tenuousness of life doesn't leave once you've discovered it. One day it's front and centre in your life, the next day off to the side. Sometimes it resides in the back recesses of your mind. But it is always accessible to you. Deep in your soul, you know that life is fleeting, and as change and challenges come your way, it is up to you to look for the joy and possibilities contained within each new day.

When cancer struck, all you wanted was to get back to normal. Once you reach the Reflection stage of recovery you realize that there's a new normal, one that involves taking an active role in the situations in your life. Having new eyes doesn't mean you're not going to get upset over rude drivers, the children arguing, or a nasty remark by a co-worker. Rather, it means seeking moments of delight despite the obstacles to joy that daily life may send your way.

> *"I wanted to keep my healthy diet, continue going to yoga classes and stick to making time for my painting class. But now I'm back to my busy life once again, and I don't always find the time to eat well or go to yoga class. I paint whenever I can, which isn't often these days. Some days it frightens me to see how far I've gone away from my initial plan for healing. I felt good then, I miss it; I need to find my way back to it."*
> — Gretta, 47 years old, ovarian cancer, 2-year survivor

As Buddha said, "It doesn't matter how long you have forgotten, only how soon you remember." (1) Many survivors talk about their desire to remember always the promises they made during treatment: to themselves, to others and/or to God. Memories of the past resurface during cancer; dreams arise, and desires are rekindled. Illness raises important exploratory questions about destiny and life's purpose. It teaches valuable lessons and offers opportunities for real change. Survivors feel the need to grasp these insights and hold onto them tightly, lest they are dimmed by time.

> *"I experience more joy in life since cancer. The work now comes in trying to keep the joy in the forefront of my life. Over time it seems to wane, and I find myself being pulled back into my old ways."*
> — Oliver, 56 years old, lung cancer, 3-year survivor

Detours will happen; they are as much a part of your journey as is following the direct route. But you can always choose to get back on the main path. Think about where you have been and what you have seen along the way. Once you have passed through all four phases of recovery and moved back into your life, in whatever form you have chosen to make of it, your final challenge is to remember.

> *"I recovered my sense of awe and wonder at the beauty of the world after I was diagnosed with cancer. Everything seems so intense now, the colours more vibrant, the smells more pungent, and the earth sweeter. I don't want to forget what I've learned."*
>
> — Casey, 28 years old, melanoma, 6-month survivor

REMEMBERING NOT TO FORGET

There is a Latin term for recalling our mortality: *memento mori*. It means "remember thy death." By keeping death foremost in your thoughts, you will also remember the sacredness of life.

In his book *Crossing the Unknown Sea*, David Whyte writes that life is about remembering, forgetting, and trying to remember again: "Remembering this life's journey beyond our present daily commute is one of life's great disciplines ... Sooner or later we forget, lose sight, we come to a place in our lives where the *vision splendid* begins to fade into the light of common day." (2) Our very future, Whyte argues, depends on finding ways to remember our original dreams and promises.

You may think you have forgotten your appreciation for every new leaf or petal because you have stopped expressing your admiration for such things on a regular basis. Before you berate yourself, consider whether your appreciation of life hasn't simply become integrated into your everyday experiences. While the voice of gratitude may seem fainter, perhaps you have developed a deeper understanding and respect for the beauty of life than you realize. But what if you have truly forgotten? What if you have veered away from your Healing Plan and let go of the things you know you need to stay well? As with the other obstacles you'll encounter, there are strategies for dealing with this situation. Here are some suggestions that have worked for other survivors:

- Start afresh
- Build in fail-safes
- Cue the memory
- Discover ritual

Start Afresh

If you feel you have lost touch with your goals for yourself, start again. Renew your Healing Plan or Vision Statement. Remind yourself about what you need to live well and feel good. Review your support people and rethink the obstacles that tend to get in your way. Sometimes time is your friend, but sometimes it can be the biggest obstacle of all.

Don't be afraid to admit that your promises have slipped away from you. It happens to many survivors. Perseverance means picking yourself up, dusting yourself off, and starting all over again.

Build in Fail-Safes

One way you can give yourself a better chance of sticking to your promises is to build change that reinforces these promises into your routine. If you promised yourself you would work less, then don't go into the office on your time off. If you promised yourself you would exercise more, hire a personal trainer or hook up with a gym buddy. It's much harder to skip a workout if you know someone is counting on you to show up. If you want to stay committed to your creative process, join a club, a class or a group that meets regularly and expects you to be there.

Support people can help you build commitment into your routine. If other people know about your intentions, they can help you fulfill them. And once you've let other people know about your plans, you are more inclined to follow through.

Another idea is to break your goal into smaller pieces. Achieve one step at a time and reward yourself at each milestone. You will build momentum and be more likely to remember your commitments as you see real progress. You can also continue with — or return to — the two daily practices. They are intended to slow you down, bring you back to the moment and remind you of the beauty that surrounds you.

Stay awake by slowing down. Change your pace enough that you can be aware of what you're experiencing even if it's uncomfortable, rather than letting your experience rush by. Whatever you're feeling, whatever you're thinking, whatever you're sensing, let the moment linger. Decelerate the rate at which you're travelling so that you can be in the now.

Cue the Memory

Many survivors use cues, keepsakes, or mementos to stay in touch with the fragility of life and the wonder of each day. They introduce one or more of these cues into their daily lives so that the cues are always present. Whenever you see a cue, it's an instant reminder of promises you've made.

> *"I wrote the promises I'd made to myself on the cover of my journal, which I keep beside my bed. I look at them every night before I go to sleep and I ask myself, 'Am I still living as if there may be no tomorrow?'"*
> — Blake, 56 years old, bladder cancer, 5-year survivor

Some other ideas include:

- taping an inspirational quote on your computer screen
- posting a photograph of your favourite outdoor setting next to the bathroom mirror
- putting a postcard on your desk from a trip you took after treatment ended
- keeping a framed photograph of yourself while in treatment
- draping a rosary or prayer beads over a door handle
- placing on your desk a rock or sea shell from a special place you've visited
- keeping a dried flower from a bouquet sent to you while you were in treatment

One survivor built a gazebo in her garden where she could retreat to smell the sweet fragrance of the various blooms in season; one kept a watch in his pocket as a tactile reminder to remain awake since time is ticking away;

another makes hundreds of origami cranes each year and says a prayer of gratitude over each one. One couple bought a painting of angels and hung it beside their bed, so that each night they would think about how fleeting life on earth is.

"My husband bought me a beautiful bracelet on the day I left the hospital. It was a reminder to both of us of the tough times and the good times we had just experienced."
— Kelly, 49 years old, lymphoma, 6-year survivor

Let's return to our puzzle metaphor for a minute. Once they've completed a complicated puzzle, some people are content with knowing that they reached their goal through effort, time, patience and perseverance, and they quietly put the puzzle away. Others want a testimony to their hard work, so they preserve their completed puzzle by laminating it, framing it, and placing it where it can be seen. What do you need to do that will help you to remember the achievements you've made through recovery and to remind you of how fast life can change?

Discover Ritual

Many survivors create a ritual that helps them celebrate life. Marking the little triumphs that dot our lives as well as the monumental ones keeps the *joie de vivre* at the centre of our lives. Some survivors throw annual parties to celebrate the blessings in their lives. The family of one survivor plants a tree every year to represent life and growth, then takes a hike together to remember the journey they shared.

"Every year I go alone to a small bed and breakfast on an island: I stay in the same room, with the same view of the Pacific Ocean, at the same time of year. I go to renew my body and replenish my spirit. I go to remember my reasons for living and to ask myself, 'Am I living the life I want to live?'"
— Mae, 62 years old, breast cancer, 9-year survivor

You can make a ritual out of any act that has meaning for you. It can happen yearly, monthly or whenever you choose. It can be done alone or in a group.

What is important in ritual is that it have symbolic meaning for you. Be creative in honouring this significant period in your life.

STAY AWAKE

As we leave you on your journey toward living the life you want to live, our wish is that you keep the questions in front of you, keep the cancer behind you, and remain awake to each moment in your life. Let the wisdom of the Sufi poet Rumi be an inspiration:

> *The breeze at dawn has secrets to tell you,*
> *Don't go back to sleep*
> *You must ask for what you really want,*
> *Don't go back to sleep.*
> *People are going back and forth across the doorsill*
> *Where the two worlds touch.*
> *The door is round and open,*
> *Don't go back to sleep* (3)

Notes

Chapter One: So, Where's the Party?

1. Glenna Halvorson-Boyd and Lisa Hunter, *Dancing in Limbo: Making Sense of Life after Cancer* (San Francisco: Jossey-Bass, 1995), p. 2.
2. Dr. Graham Smith, oncologist, personal interview, 2004.

Chapter Two: Having New Eyes

1. Marcel Proust, quoted in Dan Millman, *Sacred Journey of the Peaceful Warrior* (Tiburton, Ca.: H.J. Kramer, 1991), p. 57.
2. William Bridges, *The Way of Transition: Embracing Life's Most Difficult Moments* (Cambridge, Mass.: Perseus, 2001), p. 16.
3. C.G. Jung, *Psychological Reflections* (Princeton: Princeton University Press, 1974), p. 138.
4. Mikela Tarlow, *Navigating the Future: A Personal Guide to Achieving Success in the New Millennium* (New York: McGraw-Hill, 1999), p. 127.
5. Carol Adrienne, *When Life Changes or You Wish It Would: How to Survive and Thrive in Uncertain Times* (New York: William Morrow, 2001), p. 56.
6. Janie Brown, psychotherapist, personal interview, 2003.

Chapter Three: Laying out the Pieces

1. Michael Lerner, *Choices in Healing* (Cambridge, Mass.: MIT Press, 1998), p. 14.
2. Lance Armstrong, *It's Not about the Bike* (New York: Berkley, 2000), p. 14.
3. Joseph Campbell, *The Hero with a Thousand Faces* (Princeton: Princeton University Press, 1972).

Chapter Four: The Daily Practices

1. *American College Dictionary*, 1963 ed., s.v. "practice."
2. Kathleen Fell, nutritionist, personal interview, 2003.

Chapter Five: In Your Skin: Assessing Your Body

1. Fitzhugh Mullen, (National Coalition for Cancer Survivorship) *A Cancer Survivor's Almanac: Charting Your Journey* (Minneapolis: Chronimed Publishing, 1996).
2. Marnie McMaster, oncology nurse, personal interview, 2004.

Chapter Six: What's on Your Mind: Assessing Thoughts and Emotions

1. Jack Kornfield, *After the Ecstasy, the Laundry* (New York: Bantam, 2000), p. 36.
2. David Spiegel, *Living beyond Limits: New Hope and Help for Facing a Life-Threatening Illness* (New York: Times, 1993) p. 104.
3. Mevlâna Jalâluddîn Rumi, "The Guest House," in *The Essential Rumi*, trans. by Coleman Barks and John Moyne (New York: Harper Collins, 1985), p. 109.
4. John Milton, *Paradise Lost*, book 1, line 253.

Chapter Seven: Why Am I Here? Assessing Your Spirituality

1. Michael Lerner, *Choices in Healing* (Cambridge, Mass.: MIT Press, 1998), p. 24.
2. Rainer Maria Rilke, *Letters to a Young Poet,* trans. Joan M. Burnham (Novato: New World Library, 2000), p. 35.
3. Lis Smith, medical social worker, personal interview, 2003.
4. Alexander Solzhenitsyn, quoted in Philip Yancey, *What's So Amazing about Grace?* (Grand Rapids: Zondervan, 1997), p. 122.

Chapter Eight: Who Showed Up? Assessing Your Relationships

1. Lance Armstrong, *It's Not about the Bike* (New York: Berkley, 2001), p. 4.
2. Susan Nessim and Judith Ellis, *Cancervive: The Challenge of Life after Cancer* (Boston: Houghton Mifflin, 1991), p. 91.

Section I Conclusion: It's All Connected

1. Norman Cousins, *Anatomy of an Illness* (New York: Bantam, 1981).

Chapter Nine: Doorways to Change

1. Dr. Simon Sutcliff, oncologist and president of the British Columbia Cancer Agency, personal interview, 2004.
2. Viktor Frankl, *Man's Search for Meaning* (New York: Simon & Schuster, 1984), p. 75.
3. Pema Chödrön, *The Places That Scare You* (Boston: Shambala, 2001), p. 3.

Chapter Ten: Four Approaches to Healing: Designing a Healing Plan

1. Joseph Campbell with Bill Moyers, *The Power of Myth* (New York: Doubleday 1988), p. 92.
2. Kahlil Gibran, *The Eye of the Prophet* (Berkeley: North Atlantic, 1995).
3. Lao-Tzu, *Tao Teh Ching,* ch. 64.

Chapter Eleven: Actualizing Your Healing Plan

1. W.H. Murray, *The Scottish Himalayan Expedition* (London: Dent, 1951).

Chapter Twelve: Exploring Possibilities

1. Emily Dickinson, "I Dwell in Possibility," in *Complete Poems of Emily Dickinson,* ed. by Thomas Johnson (Boston: Little, Brown, 1960).
2. Henry David Thoreau, *Writings of Henry David Thoreau,* vol. 2 (Boston: Houghton Mifflin, 1906), p. 356.
3. Mary Oliver, "The Summer Day," in Mary Oliver, *New and Selected Poems* (Boston: Beacon, 1992), p. 94.

Chapter Thirteen: Re-Evaluating Your Healing Plan

1. Carol Adrienne, *When Life Changes or You Wish It Would: How to Survive and Thrive in Difficult Times* (New York: Harper Collins, 2002), p. 101.
2. Dan Millman, *The Laws of the Spirit* (Tiburon, Ca.: H.J. Kramer, 1995), p. 31.

Chapter Fourteen: Growth through Adversity

1. Viktor Frankl, *Man's Search for Meaning* (New York: Simon & Schuster, 1959), p. 76.
2. Aldous Huxley, introduction to *Texts and Pretexts* (London: Chatto & Windus, 1932).
3. Lance Armstrong, *It's Not about the Bike* (New York: Berkley, 2000), p. 284.
4. St. Augustine, quoted in Helen Waddell, *The Desert Fathers* (Ann Arbor: University of Michigan Press, 1957), p. 24.
5. Viktor Frankl, *Man's Search for Meaning* (New York: Simon & Schuster, 1959).
6. Carlos Castaneda, anecdote quoted in George Cappannelli and Sedena Cappannelli, *Authenticity* (Cincinnati: Emmis Books, 2004), p. 119.
7. M. Scott Peck, *Further along the Road Less Travelled* (New York: Simon & Schuster, 1993), p. 49.

Chapter Fifteen: From Wounds to Wisdom

1. Melody Beattie, *Choices: Taking Control of Your Life and Making It Matter* (New York: Harper Collins, 2002), p. 112.
2. Kat Duff, *The Alchemy of Illness* (New York: Bell Tower, 1993), p. 43.
3. Pema Chödrön, *When Things Fall Apart: Heart Advice for Difficult Times* (Boston: Shambhala, 1997), p. 93.
4. Mevlâna Jalâluddîn Rumi, "Out beyond Ideas," in *The Essential Rumi*, trans. Coleman Barks and John Moyne (New York: Harper Collins, 1985), p. 36.

Chapter Sixteen: Living with Uncertainty

1. D.H. Lawrence, *Late Essays and Articles* (Cambridge: Cambridge University Press, 2004), p. 219.
2. William Bridges, *The Way of Transition: Embracing Life's Most Difficult Moments* (Cambridge, Mass.: Perseus , 2001), p. 69.
3. Dr. Lee Pulos, psychologist, personal interview, 2003.
4. Jack Kornfield, *A Path with Heart* (New York: Bantam, 1993).
5. Michelle Tocher, *How to Ride a Dragon* (Toronto: Key Porter, 2002), p. 152.

Chapter Seventeen: Don't Go Back to Sleep

1. Buddha, quoted in Stephen Levine, *A Year to Live* (New York: Bell Tower, 1997), p. 8.
2. David Whyte, *Crossing the Unknown Sea* (New York: Riverhead, 2001) p. 70.
3. Mevlâna Jalâluddîn Rumi, "Don't Go Back to Sleep," in *Open Secret: Versions of Rumi*, trans. John Moyne and Coleman Barks (Boston: Shambala, 1984).

Resources

BOOKS

Cancer Survivorship

Armstrong, Lance. *It's Not about the Bike*. New York: Berkley, 2000.
An inspirational autobiography by a well-known sports hero and cancer survivor.

Halvorson-Boyd, Glenna, and Lisa K. Hunter. *Dancing in Limbo: Making Sense of Life after Cancer*. San Francisco: Jossey-Bass, 1995.
Inspiration, affirmation and informative insights into life after cancer from two survivors.

Harpham, Wendy S. *After Cancer: A Guide to Your New Life*. New York: W.W. Norton, 1994.
A thorough description of the physical, emotional and social after-effects of cancer, from a physician and survivor.

National Coalition for Cancer Survivorship. *A Cancer Survivor's Almanac: Charting Your Journey*. Hoboken: John Wiley, 2004.
Straightforward and compassionate, written by a number of professionals who have defined the survivorship movement from the beginning.

Nessim, Susan, and Judith Ellis. *Cancervive: The Challenge of Life after Cancer*. Boston: Houghton Mifflin, 2000.
Inspiring and practical. Susan is the founder of Cancervive, a support group for survivors.

Schnipper, Hester. *After Breast Cancer: A Common-Sense Guide to Life after Treatment*. New York: Bantam, 2003.
A useful guide for women who are beginning their recovery process. Schnipper writes from a professional and personal view.

Tocher, Michelle. *How to Ride a Dragon*. Toronto: Key Porter, 2002.
A beautifully crafted weaving of mythology, narrative and the voices of breast cancer survivors.

Change and Transition Management

Adrienne, Carol. *When Life Changes or You Wish It Would: How to Survive and Thrive in Uncertain Times*. New York: Harper Collins, 2002.
Warm and accessible style, acknowledging that change can be both exhilarating and terrifying.

Beattie, Melody. *Choices: Taking Control of Your Life & Making It Matter.* New York: Harper Collins, 2002
  Uses personal stories and inspirational prose to help navigate through the everyday choices, and to find hope in times of despair.

Bridges, William. *Transitions: Making Sense of Life's Changes.* Reading, Mass.: Addison-Wesley, 1980.
  An in-depth exploration, offering suggestions for navigating in order to better handle change.

Bridges, William. *The Way of Transition: Embracing Life's Most Difficult Moments.* Cambridge, Mass.: Perseus, 2001.
  Beautifully written and uplifting; the author describes his own journey through a serious life transition.

Perkins-Reed, Marcia. *Thriving in Transition: Effective Living in Times of Change.* New York: Touchstone, 1996.
  A practical and holistic approach to negotiating change.

Senge, Peter, Art Kleiner, Charlotte Roberts, Richard B. Ross, and Bryan J. Ross. *The Fifth Discipline Fieldbook.* New York: Doubleday, 1994.
  While this book presents strategies for building a learning organization, many of the prinicples are relevant for addressing personal change.

Senge, Peter, Art Kleiner, Charlotte Roberts, Richard B. Ross, and Bryan J. Ross. *The Dance of Change: Challenges to Sustaining Momentum in Learning Organizations.* New York: Doubleday, 1999.
  Despite its business focus, this book offers valuable direction on how to achieve permanent and sustainable change.

Spencer, Sabrina, and John Adams. *Life Change: Growing through Personal Transitions.* California: Impact Publishers, 1990.
  Describes a variety of life's inevitable transitions and presents a seven-stage approach to dealing with change.

Loss and Grief Resources

Boulanger, Gail. *Life Goes On: Losing, Letting Go and Living Again.* Nanoose Bay, B.C., Canada: Notch Hill Books, 2002.

Deits, Bob. *Life after Loss: A Practical Guide to Renewing Your Life after Experiencing Major Loss.* Lifelong Books, 2004.

Kubler-Ross, Elisabeth, and David Kessler. *Life Lessons.* New York: Scribner, 2000.

Levine, Stephen. *Unattended Sorrow: Recovering from Loss and Reviving the Heart.* Emmaus: Rodale, 2005.

Powning, Beth. *The Hat Box Letters.* Toronto: Knopf Canada, 2005.

Siebert, Al. *The Resiliency Advantage: Master Change, Thrive under Pressure, and Bounce Back from Setbacks.* San Francisco: Berrett-Koehler, 2005.

Complementary Medicine
American Cancer Society. *American Cancer Society's Guide to Complementary and Alternative Cancer Methods.* Atlanta, G.: American Cancer Society, 2000.
A comprehensive guide to traditional and complementary therapies.

Gordon, James S, and Sharon Curtin. *Comprehensive Cancer Care: Integrating Alternative, Complementary, and Conventional Therapies.* Cambridge, Mass.: Perseus, 2001.
A thorough guide to evaluating and choosing treatments and practitioners.

Lerner, Michael. *Choices in Healing.* Cambridge, Mass.: MIT Press, 1996.
A compelling and medically sound guidebook to conventional and alternative practices.

Inspirational
Bolen, Jean Shinoda. *Close to the Bone.* New York: Simon & Schuster, 1996.
Combining psychiatric medical experience with myth and spirituality, the author explores the impact of serious illess.

Chödrön, Pema. *When Things Fall Apart.* Boston: Shambhala, 2002.
An American Buddhist nun gives compassionate advice and teaches how to move through painful situations with curiosity and kindness.

Kabat-Zinn, John. *Wherever You Go, There You Are.* New York: Hyperion, 1994.
The author maps out a simple path for awakening to wisdom and cultivating mindfulness.

Kornfield, Jack. *A Path with Heart.* New York: Bantam, 1989.
A practical approach to meditation and spiritual development, using stories from his own experience to illuminate the path of a more general spiritual journey

Kornfield, Jack. *After the Ecstasy, the Laundry.* New York: Bantam, 2000.
Buddhist teacher and internationally known meditation master draws upon his own story as well as the experiences of leaders of other faith-based traditions to help understand how a modern spiritual journey unfolds.

Millman, Dan. *The Laws of Spirit*. Tiburon, Ca.: H.J. Kramer, 1995.
A beautifully written story with wise and playful teachings about everyday life decisions.

Oliver, Mary. *New and Selected Poems*. Boston: Beacon Press, 1992.
Renowned poet who inspires and provides insights into life's meaning.

Salzberg, Sharon. *Faith: Trusting Your Own Deepest Experience*. New York: Riverhead, 2002.
Renowned meditation teacher helps face the unknown, offering insights into faith as a healing quality and learning to trust your inner voice.

Thich Nhat Hanh. *Peace Is Every Step*. New York: Bantam, 1992.
World-renowned Zen master shows how to make positive use of everyday situations and help find peace.

Tolle, Eckhart. *The Power of Now*. Vancouver, B.C.: Namaste, 1997.
An easy-to-read spiritual guide on how to derive strength and a sense of peace from the present.

Whyte, David. *Crossing the Unknown Sea: Work as a Pilgrimage of Identity*. New York: Riverhead, 2001.
Inspirational, written by a poet who provides mesmerizing stories and insights aimed to help you take steps toward your true goals

ORGANIZATIONS AND INTERNET

Cancer Information Services
The following is a partial listing of the many excellent resources available. These are well-established websites that have links or resource pages for more extensive information.

American Cancer Society (ACS)
1599 Clifton Road, NE
Atlanta, GA 30329
1-800-ACS-2345
www.cancer.org
Focus: community support services, resources, information, research and advocacy.

Canadian Cancer Society (CCS)
10 Alcorn Avenue, Suite 200
Toronto, ON M4V 3B1
416-961-7223 or Information Services 1-888-939-3333.
www.cancer.ca
Focus: community support services, resources, information, research and advocacy.

American Institute for Cancer Research (AICR)
1759 R Street, NW
Washington, DC 20009
202-328-7744 or 1-800-843-8114
www.aicr.org
Focus: nutritional information, nutritional hotline, support network, information and resources.

American Psychosocial Oncology Society (APOS)
2365 Hunters Way
Charlottesville, VA 22911
434-293-5350 or 1-866-276-7443
www.apos-society.org
Focus: referrals to local counselling and support services throughout United States. Educational programs, research and advocacy work.

American Society of Clinical Oncology (ASCO)
1900 Duke Street, Suite 200
Alexandria, VA 22314
703-299-0150
www.asco.org
Focus: comprehensive patient support organization list, scientific and educational programs.

People Living with Cancer
www.plwc.org
Focus: information on more than 50 types of cancer and their treatments, clinical trials, side effects and coping. Includes live chats, message boards and links to support groups.

Association of Cancer Online Resources (ACOR)
www.acor.org
Focus: un-moderated online discussion lists for patients, family, friends, researchers and physicians.

Cancer Care, Inc.
275 Seventh Avenue
New York, NY 10001
1-800-813-4673
www.cancercare.org
Focus: free professional support through counselling, education, information and financial assistance.

Candlelighters Childhood Cancer Foundation
1-800-366-2223
www.candlelighters.org
Focus: a network of support for children, parents and caregivers in USA.

Candlelighters Childhood Cancer Foundation of Canada
416-489-6440 or 1-800-363-1062
www.candlelighter.ca
   Focus: a network of support for children, parents and caregivers in Canada.

Commonweal Cancer Help Program
P.O. Box 316
Bolinas, CA 94924
415-868-0970
www.commonweal.org
   Focus: non-profit health and environment research institute that conducts residential
   retreats for people living with cancer.

Gilda's Club, INC.
322 Eighth Avenue, Suite 1402
New York, NY 10001
917-305-1200 or 888-GILDA-4-U
www.gildasclub.org
   Focus: support for cancer patients, their families, and friends, including workshops, net-
   working and children's program.

Lance Armstrong Foundation
P.O. Box 161150
Austin, TX 78716-1150
512-236-8820
www.laf.org
LIVE**STRONG** Survivor*Care* resource program
1-866-235-7205
www.livestrong.org
   Focus: information, education, counselling services, and referrals to other resources for
   cancer survivors.

Planet Cancer
www.planetcancer.org
   Focus: online forum and support community for young adults with cancer, information on camps, established support groups and informal gatherings.

National Cancer Institute (NCI)
31 Center Drive
Bethesda, MD 20892
301-435-3848 or 1-800-422-6237
NCI is a constituent of the National Institute of Health (NIH)
www.nci.nih.gov
www.cancer.gov

National Cancer Institute, Office of Cancer Survivorship (OCS)
6116 Executive Boulevard, Suite 404
Bethesda, MD 20892-7397
301-402-2964

www.survivorship.cancer.gov
   Focus: educational publications and resources, promote survivorship research.

www.nci.nih.gov
www.cancer.gov
   Focus: information, educational resources, cancer information service and research.

National Cancer Institute of Canada (NCIC)
10 Alcorn Avenue, Suite 200
Toronto, ON M4V 3B1
416-961-7223
www.ncic.cancer.ca
   Focus: information, educational resources and cancer research.

National Coalition for Cancer Survivorship (NCCS)
1010 Wayne Avenue, Suite 770
Silver Spring, MD 20910
1-877-622-7937
www.canceradvocacy.org
www.cancersurvivaltoolbox.org
   Focus: survivorship information, resources and advocacy.

National Center for Complementary and Alternative Medicine (NCCAM)
P.O. Box 7923
Gaithersburg, MD 20898-7923
1-866-644-6226
www.nccam.nih.gov
   Focus: information about the safety and effectiveness of complementary and alternative medicine practices.

National Childhood Cancer Foundation (NCCF)
CureSearch
Headquarters Office
4600 East West Highway #60
Bethesda, MD 20814-3457
240-235-2200 or 1-800-458-6223
www.curesearch.org
   Focus: information on childhood cancer for patients, families and health care professionals.

National Family Caregivers Association
10400 Connecticut Avenue, Suite 500
Kensington, MD 20895-3944
301-942-6430 or 1-800-896-3650
www.nfcacares.org
   Focus: advocacy organization with tips and statistics on caregiving.

Caregivers, Inc.
1-800-829-2734
www.caregiver.com
   Focus: online newsletter, workshops, and information on caregiving topics.

The Ulman Cancer Fund for Young Adults
5575 Sterrett Place, Suite 340A
Columbia, MD 21044
410-964-0202 or 1-800-393-FUND (3863)
www.ulmanfund.org
 Focus: support, education and resources for young adults with cancer, their families
 and friends.

The Wellness Community (National)
919 18th Street, NW, Suite 54
Washington, DC 2006
202-659-9709 or 1-888-793-WELL (1-888-793-9355)
www.wellness-community.org
 Focus: emotional support, educational programs, exercise, nutrition and relaxation
 workshops.

Wellspring
81 Wellesley Street East
Toronto, ON M4Y 1H6
416-961-1928
www.wellspring.ca
 Focus: free support programs to individuals and their families living with cancer.

Breast Cancer Information Services
Canadian Breast Cancer Network (CBCN)
300 – 331 Cooper Street
Ottawa, ON K2P 0G5
613-230-3044 / 1-800-685-8820
www.cbcn.ca

Living Beyond Breast Cancer
10 East Athens Avenue, Suite 204
Ardmore, PA 19003
610-645-4567 or 888-753-5222
www.lbbc.org
 Focus: information and support, conferences on survivorship issues.

National Alliance of Breast Cancer Organizations (NABCO)
9 East 37th Street, 10th Floor
New York, NY 10016
212-889-0606 or 888-806-2226
www.nabco.org
 Focus: information and resources, support group listings. They publish an annual breast
 cancer resource book.

The Susan G. Komen Breast Cancer Foundation
5005 LBJ Freeway, Suite 250
Dallas, TX 75244
975-855-1600 or 800-I'M-AWARE (helpline)
www.komen.org
   Focus: community-based outreach programs, educational materials, resources and support programs information.

Y-Me National Breast Cancer Organization
212 West Van Buren Street, Suite 1000
Chicago, IL 60607
312-986-8338
www.y-me.org
24-hour toll-free hotline with trained peer counselors:
English: 1-800-221-2141 / Spanish: 1-800-986-9505
   Focus: support services, information and advocacy.

Young Survival Coalition
155 6th Avenue, 10th floor
New York, NY 10013
212-206-6610
www.youngsurvival.org
   Focus: educational programs, annual conference, advocacy and awareness for young women living with breast cancer.

National Lymphedema Network
1611 Telegraph Avenue, Suite 1111
Oakland, CA 94612
1-800-541-3259
www.lymphnet.org
   Focus: lymphedema prevention and management.

Other Specific Cancer Sites
Brain Tumor Foundation of Canada
1-800-265-5106.
www.braintumor.ca
   Focus: free printed and online information as well as access to support groups.

National Brain Tumor Foundation
22 Battery Street, Suite 612
San Francisco, CA 94111-5520
1-800-934-CURE (1-800-934-2873)
www.braintumor.org
   Focus: conferences, website, printed information, patient information line, patient and caregiver support network.

Colorectal Cancer Association of Canada
60 St. Clair Avenue East, Suite 204
Toronto, ON M4T 1N5
416-920-4333 or 1-888-318-9442
www.ccac-accc.ca
  Focus: support, education, and resource links.

Canadian Kidney Foundation
300 – 5165 Sherbrooke Street West
Montréal, QC H4A 1T6
514-369-4806 or 1-800-361-7494
www.kidney.ca
  Focus: information and support to help adapt to the challenges of living with kidney
  disease.

Kidney Cancer Association
1-800-850-236-8820
www.kidneycancerassociation.org
  Focus: support and educational information.

Canadian Lung Association
1-888-566-LUNG (5864)
www.lung.ca
  Focus: information and links to lung cancer support and advocacy groups.

Lung Cancer Alliance
1- 800-298-2436 (US only); 202-463-2080
www.lungcanceralliance.org
  Focus: dedicated solely to helping those living with lung cancer improve the quality of
  their lives through advocacy, support, and education.

Gynaecologic Cancer Foundation
230 West Monroe, Suite 2528
Chicago, IL 60606 USA

312-578-1439 or 1-800-444-4441
www.wcn.org/gcf
  Focus: any cancer related to female reproductive tract: ovary, endometrium, cervix,
  vulva and vagina.

Canadian Prostate Cancer Network (CPCN)
P.O. Box 1253
Lakefield, ON K0L 2H0
705- 652-9200 or 1-866-810-CPCN (2726)
  Focus: support groups and educational resources.

Canadian Leukemia and Lymphoma Society
172 King Street East, Suite 305

Oshawa, ON L1H 1B7
416-661-9541
www.lls.org/canada
Focus: comprehensive services to patients and families touched by blood cancers.

Melanoma International Foundation
250 Mapleflower Road
Glenmoore, PA 19343
1-866-463-6663
www.melanomainternational.org
Focus: information and resources related to melanoma.

Support for People with Oral and Head and Neck Cancer (SPOHNC)
P.O. Box 53
Locust Valley, NY 11560-0053
1-800-377-0928
www.spohnc.org
Focus: oral cancer and cancers of the head and neck.

Testicular Cancer Links
www.tc.ca.com
Focus: web access to multiple other links related to testicular cancer.

Thyroid Cancer Survivors' Association (THYCA)
1-877-588-7904
www.thyca.org
Focus: current information, support services, and resources on survivors' issues.

American Foundation for Urologic Disease (AFUD)
1128 North Charles Street
Baltimore, MD 21201
1-800-242-2383
www.afud.org
Focus: access to various health sites providing information on urologic diseases and/or conditions.

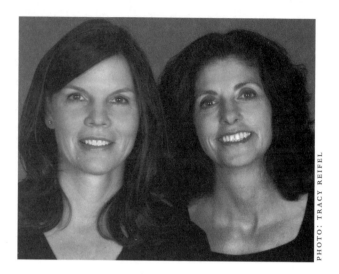

SHERRI MAGEE was personally affected by cancer when five members of her family were diagnosed with the disease. This inspired her to pursue a Ph.D. in order to understand the short- and long-term effects of cancer and its treatment on those who survived. For over fifteen years she has designed personal cancer recovery programs for family, friends and clients and has trained physiotherapists, exercise specialists and personal trainers to work with cancer survivors in a variety of settings. Sherri chaired the International Cancer Rehabilitation Conference several times and is a frequent speaker at medical and educational conferences. She is the co-founder of the hugely successful "Abreast in a Boat" dragon boat society, past Executive Director of the Hope House Cancer Centre, and an honourary clinical instructor at the University of British Columbia's School of Rehabilitation Sciences.

KATHY SCALZO is president of a Vancouver based consulting group specializing in change and transition planning and management. She obtained her Masters degree in Organizational Development from Pepperdine University. Over the last twenty years, she has worked with individuals as well as over 200 health care organizations, government departments and non-profit agencies. She has extensive experience as a consultant and seminar leader across Canada and is a frequent speaker at professional and educational conferences. For nine years, she was a core faculty member of the Canadian Medical Association's Physician Management Institute, which provides physicians with training in conflict resolution and change management. She is an honourary clinical instructor at the University of British Columbia's School of Rehabilitation Sciences.